THE GOOD NEWS EATING PLAN FOR TYPE II DIABETES

Elaine Magee, M.P.H., R.D.

John Wiley & Sons, Inc.

New York • Chichester • Weinheim • Brisbane • Singapore • Toronto

Library of Congress Cataloging-in-Publication Data

Magee, Elaine.
    The good news eating plan for type II diabetes / Elaine Magee.
        p.   cm.
    Includes index.
    ISBN 0-471-17624-9 (pbk. : alk. paper)
    1. Non-insulin-dependent diabetes—Diet therapy.   I. Title.
RC662.M332   1998
616.4'620654—dc21   97-38639

Printed in the United States of America

10 9 8 7 6 5 4 3 2 1

THE GOOD NEWS
EATING PLAN FOR
TYPE II DIABETES

This book is dedicated to all the people I know and love with Type II diabetes: my father, Don Moquette; my sister-in-law, Chris Magee; my favorite teacher, Sharon Belshaw-Jones; and my friend Mike Nielsen.

CONTENTS

Foreword   xi
Acknowledgments   xiii

INTRODUCTION   1

Why Did *I* Write This Book?   1
What's It All About?   3

PART ONE
WHAT YOU NEED TO KNOW TO MANAGE YOUR DIABETES   5

1   YOUR HEALTH CARE
    TEAM   7

The Three Keys to Success   7
How to Build a Health Care Team   8
Your Health Care Team: What to Expect on Your First Visit   9
Other Members of Your Health Care Team   15
And Don't Forget Your Family   16
Once Again, the Good News   16

2   GOOD NEWS FOR THOSE WHO
    ENJOY EATING   17

The Buddy System: Pairing Carbohydrates
    with Fat or Protein   18
High-Carbohydrate, High-Fiber Foods—at Every Meal   19
Mono- versus Polyunsaturated Fat   22
Sugar Is No Longer Taboo   25
How Sweet It Is: The Latest on Alternative Sweeteners   26
Eat, Drink, and Be Merry?   30
Ten to Twenty Pounds May Be All You Have to Lose   31

3 NEW DIET GUIDELINES FROM
THE AMERICAN DIABETES ASSOCIATION   33

Two Great Reasons to Eat Well   33
General Recommendations and New Perspectives   34
How Much Is Right for *Most*   37

4 NUTRITION GOALS AND
STRATEGIES   42

Goal #1   Controlling Blood Glucose Levels   43
Goal #2   Normalizing Blood Lipid Levels   49
Strategy #1:   Moderate Weight Loss   55
Strategy #2:   Cutting Calories   60
Are You Overeating?   61
Strategy #3:   Exercise   62
Strategy #4:   Eating Smaller, More Frequent Meals   64
Attitude Adjustment: Getting Your Mind Right   65

PART TWO

THE GOOD NEWS EATING PLAN   67

5 THE C-F-F GRAM-COUNTING
PLAN   69

Portion Size Success   70
Counting Carbohydrates   74
Counting Fat   76
Counting Fiber   77
Considering Calories   78
Carbo-Counting When on Insulin   80
Combination Foods   83
Be Your Own Blood Glucose Detective I   83

6   ALL THE ADVICE AND DATA YOU NEED
    TO MANAGE YOUR DIET   107

    Being Your Own Blood Glucose Detective II:
        The Diet Diary   108
    The Glycemic Index Guide   110
    Timing Your Medication and Meals   119
    How to Stop Bad Snacking Habits   119
    Free Foods for Any Time of Day (or Night) 121
    Free and Almost-Free Recipes   122
    More on Monounsaturated and Saturated Fat 124
    Americanizing the Mediterranean Diet   124
    Making Fiber Your Friend   127
    Do the Math   132
    Mealtime Tips—Breakfast   133
    Mealtime Tips—Lunch   136
    Mealtime Tips—Dinner   137
    Solving the Dining-Out Dilemma   137
    Take It One Step at a Time   150
    Diabetic by Marriage   151

7   SUPERMARKET SCORE CARD—THE BEST BETS FOR
    DISCRIMINATING PEOPLE WITH DIABETES   152

    Does No Sugar Mean Bad Flavor?   152
    Reading Labels   153
    Rating the "No-Sugar" and "Less-Sugar" Products for
        Taste and Nutrition   155
    The Winner's Circle of Light Products   164

8   RECIPES YOU NEED AND RECIPES
    YOU ASKED FOR   177

    Index   215

FOREWORD

It would be nice if diabetes were a single entity and its treatment were cut-and-dried. But diabetes is a chameleon, manifesting itself differently in different people and even changing throughout its course within the same person. This means that diabetes, especially Type II diabetes, demands an arsenal of treatments. There is no one dietary approach, no one medication or dose, and no one activity that suits everyone with diabetes.

As if the diagnosis itself were not enough, this confusing array of options complicates treatment decisions. The good news is that all of these options exist. As a person with Type I diabetes, I have said for years that "an optionist is by nature an optimist." Youwould not want to be locked into only one treatment approach. What if you were the one exception to that rule or treatment? You'd want the opportunity to try something else. When you have options, *you* don't have to blame yourself if something doesn't work; it simply means *that* option wasn't right for you.

Elaine Magee has done the job of taking the many confusing options for meal planning for Type II diabetes and melded them into one commonsense, cohesive plan. That plan is the "carbohydrate-fat-fiber" approach. Too often, people with Type II diabetes are taught about these components in isolation from one another.

And yet, this approach can still be adapted for all individuals with diabetes, when they see their dietician or diabetes educator. Moreover, Elaine has enlisted the help of people with diabetes to taste-test the best fast food, restaurant choices, and healthy food products on the market. With the legwork already done for you, you can set your mind to the meal plan and pay attention to your blood sugar control instead of wading through the many choices available in the grocery store.

I invite you to enjoy this book, which will lead you to enjoy your health. The ultimate gift for anyone with diabetes is to approach life as if he or she did not have diabetes. A large part of that experience is to eat the foods you've always enjoyed . . . and now, you can!

—Susan L. Thom, R.D., C.D.E.
Marketing Manager for Diabetes Disease State Management
for Boehringer Mannheim Corporation
1994–1995 President of the American Association of
Diabetes Educators

ACKNOWLEDGMENTS

I deeply appreciate the diligence of Susan Thom, past president of the American Association of Diabetes Educators, who took time out of her very hectic schedule to review the book and write the foreword. And this book would never have gotten off the ground without the many wonderful people in diabetes support groups who let me visit their meetings and who took the time to answer my questionnaire and express their questions and concerns. I thought of you all as I wrote this book.

INTRODUCTION

If you have Type II (adult onset) diabetes, or have a family member who does, you've found a book that will help you eat better and stay healthier.

Type II people are all too used to doctors handing them a sample menu and sending them off with a not-so-fond farewell of "just lose the weight." Complicated drug and diet treatment orders are quickly dictated to you in an often rushed fifteen-minute session. No, people with diabetes definitely *don't* need someone else authoritatively lecturing on the limits of the diabetic diet or threatening them with a long list of possible complications.

What you *do* need is a good friend, well versed in food and nutrition, who will help you make sense of the situation. Someone who understands what you are going through. Someone who will consider your diet and lifestyle preferences. I'm going to be that friend for you, a partner in your treatment, a contributor to your health care team. Together we will find an eating plan that you can not only live with, but love! One that is just right for you.

Let me tell you about your new friend and how this book came to be.

WHY DID *I* WRITE THIS BOOK?

You've heard the expression, "You can lead a horse to water but you can't make him drink?" I have been dragging my Type II father (whom I love dearly) to the water for years, and . . . well, he's not drinking. Oh sure, every now and then he might sip the water a little, or dip his big toe in to test the temperature. But when it comes right down to it, he's not drinking. He has had diabetes since 1983, but he hasn't yet bought into the idea of changing the way he eats and exercises to manage his blood sugar better. His unwillingness to change is probably bigger than his will to live longer and to feel better.

In my last-ditch effort to help my father with his diabetes, I began read-

1

ing journal articles and attending seminars on diabetes. This wasn't too hard, since I am a registered dietitian who writes books and a newspaper column. Around the same time quite a few people urged me to write a book for people with diabetes, claiming there weren't any "good" books out there to help them tie different kinds of information together. I visited my father's diabetes support group and witnessed firsthand how these wonderful people were struggling with the food/diet portion of their diabetes therapy.

I wanted to try to help the people who were already at the water trough, to strain the metaphor a bit further, though not always happy with what was there to drink. My hope was that by helping them, I might also help my dad and several other Type II people in my life. My favorite teacher, who has continued to inspire me with her creative energy since I took her eighth grade drama class, has had Type II diabetes for years now. My sister-in-law and a close friend, both in their thirties, recently had to adjust to developing this disease. My first wish is that these special people, and all other Type IIs, can live long, healthful, and happy lives with diabetes.

Admittedly my interest in Type II diabetes isn't entirely altruistic. I also wanted to know all there is to know it so *I* could better prevent the disease in me and my daughters, now that diabetes is in the family tree. So my second wish is that many people at risk for Type II diabetes might prevent it from progressing by eating and exercising defensively and maintaining their "fighting weight" through the years.

To make these wishes come true, we have a lot of work to do. But I think you'll enjoy the challenge and the results.

Even before you have a game plan, you have to have a team. In the first chapter of the book, I tell you how to put together a health care team, with you as captain. I introduce the three keys to successfully managing diabetes: monitoring, exercising regularly, and following your own personalized eating plan. In the next two chapters, I provide a wealth of nutrition information, including some good news about what you can eat. In chapter 4, I cover important health and diet issues and offer strategies for reaching your nutritional goals.

The first four chapters make up Part One, What You Need to Know to Manage Your Diabetes. The second four constitute Part Two, The Good News Eating Plan. In chapter 5, I detail the carbohydrates-fat-fiber gram counting plan, including all the data you'll need. What isn't there is in chapter 6: the glycemic index of foods and tips for low-fat, high-fiber eating at home and while dining out. In chapter 7, I go with you to the supermarket and rate dozens of no- and low-sugar products. Finally, in chapter 8, I share nearly fifty recipes that are both tasty and satisfying and that will help you meet your nutritional goals. I also include several dessert items requested by my father's diabetes support group.

WHAT'S IT ALL ABOUT?

Managing your diabetes entails glucose monitoring, exercise, and the right diet plan for you. I'll explain how to pick a health care team to assist you in using these three keys to success, and I'll provide all the information and guidance I can to make the third key (eating) as easy, healthful, and enjoyable as possible.

The good news is you can eat better, be healthier, and still love food. Read on and enjoy.

PART ONE

WHAT YOU NEED TO KNOW TO MANAGE YOUR DIABETES

1

YOUR HEALTH CARE TEAM

For those with Type II diabetes, I have good—perhaps *very* good—news and what some of you might consider bad news. The bad news is that your treatment is going to get more complicated. The good news is that your daily life should become a lot more pleasant, satisfying, and even fun. Why? Because you'll be eating more enjoyable (and safer) meals. And you should be feeling better, too.

These changes are a result of the emerging trend toward more individuality and flexibility in the care of diabetes. That is, your daily treatment will be adapted to your own personal needs and medical condition. Sounds good, and it is. The complicating factor is that you must be actively involved in the ongoing decision-making process. You will be a vital member of your health care team. In fact (now don't alarm the doctor), you'll be team captain.

And why shouldn't you be in charge? Ultimately, the success of your treatment lies in your day-to-day lifestyle decisions, because you provide 95 to 99 percent of your own care. The critical elements of care—namely, keeping track of your blood sugar, eating right, and exercising—are in your hands.

Now, that doesn't mean you have to do everything or know everything. You will, however, have to coordinate the contributions of the medical experts that are available to help you and to make the decisions that affect your life. Let's see how that works by examining what I call the three keys to successful diabetes management.

THE THREE KEYS TO SUCCESS

Many diabetes specialists believe there are three keys to successfully managing diabetes: (1) monitoring your blood glucose levels, (2) exercising regularly, and (3) following your personalized eating plan—all according to your health care team's advice. The three keys work together, and each is essential.

7

Keeping your blood glucose as near normal as possible protects your body from diabetic complications further down the line. Certainly, regularly measuring your blood glucose is a necessary step toward tightly controlling your blood sugar. Your health care team can work with you on fine-tuning your health care plan (including adjusting medications, changing your eating plan, and modifying exercise programs) if they know how your blood sugar is being affected from day to day. Regular monitoring also helps you focus mentally on staying with your personalized treatment plan.

Creating and sticking with your own specially tailored exercise program also makes you stay on target. Besides helping to control blood glucose levels, exercise improves the cardiovascular system, thus reducing the risk of heart disease, and aids in weight loss, which can have significant benefits for people with diabetes. An exercise physiologist can work with you on finding the types of exercises that best suit your body and your interests. You might put together routines that combine a variety of activities, from walking to country-western dancing, from swimming to riding a stationary bike. Look for things you can do, and that you *will* do because you enjoy them, and that provide the benefits—and safety—you need. Exercise physiologists have the technical training to help tailor a program that will be right for you.

Finally, good diabetes control cannot be achieved without meal planning. A registered dietitian (preferably one who is also a certified diabetes educator, C.D.E.) can work with you to put together a personalized eating plan that will incorporate your health goals as well as your personal preferences for meal times, food choices, and lifestyle needs.

Your personalized eating plan may encourage your body to lose weight slowly (or maintain your weight) if that is one of your treatment goals. It is also designed to match your medical treatment closely should you need to take insulin or other medications. And just as with regular monitoring and exercise, adhering to a personalized eating plan enhances your chances of successfully managing your diabetes, because you are more likely to stick with a plan that you helped design and with which you are comfortable and even happy.

With these keys to success in mind, let's talk about how to get the expert help you need.

HOW TO BUILD A HEALTH CARE TEAM

If you've been dealing with Type II diabetes for a while and/or you are not blessed with great health insurance and first-rate, readily available medical treatment, you're likely to be a bit skeptical about captaining your own health care team. And you're right to be. Today, many of us have to fight for good health care. And when something beyond the long-accepted and traditional approach is sought by a patient, the obstacles only increase.

Your personal physician, for instance, may not be up to date on the recent scientific evidence indicating that keeping blood sugar as close to normal ("tight control") can significantly reduce the complications of diabetes. But many researchers do, in fact, support tight control of blood sugar through intense diet counseling, monitoring, and exercise programs. The American Diabetes Association now supports that point of view. (And we'll discuss that significant development in chapter 3.) However, some physicians may not be willing to march in that direction just yet.

It is also quite possible that your physician may not be willing to work on a more intensive treatment plan because she doesn't have the time or isn't reimbursed for these additional efforts. Perhaps there isn't a system in place for your physician to work closely with other professionals who will be able to help you with an eating or exercise plan.

Whatever the reasons, you may have to become your own advocate. By reading this book, you are demonstrating the willingness to learn and gaining the knowledge to do just that. You may have to spend your own money to see an exercise specialist, a dietitian who is specially trained in diabetes, and/or a certified diabetes educator. (The C.D.E. is specially trained to counsel diabetics on every aspect of self-care.) You may also have to spend your own time to find these people. Ask around in your diabetes support group for recommendations. (If you don't belong to a support group, think about joining one. If there isn't a group in your area, consider starting one.)

Your personal physician should be willing to provide the support you want also. If he/she isn't regularly conducting the screening tests described below, request that he/she do so. And even if he/she is performing the tests, you may have to ask (insist on) the numbers, so you know exactly where you stand. And if you can't seem to get your doctor on board, consider looking for one who will fit into your team. Remember, your health and your life are at stake.

YOUR HEALTH CARE TEAM: WHAT TO EXPECT ON YOUR FIRST VISIT

Before you read the long list of shoulds below, remember that your first visit needs to be very comprehensive. Most other visits to your physician will be much shorter. Incidentally, these recommendations assume you're starting with a new doctor who is open to intensive, patient-oriented treatment. However, if you are reinventing your relationship with your old physician, please modify the advice to fit your situation.

Your doctor, or other health care team members in his/her office, should ask questions about your life, complications, and any diabetes treatments you've had before seeing her. For example, she should want to know about any infections you've had, complications that resulted, and subsequent treatments. She needs to know what medicines you are currently taking and whether you smoke, have high blood pressure, or have a family history of heart disease. She should ask you questions about your current diet and exercise habits. It is also helpful for her to know what other medical problems you've had and if anyone else in your family has diabetes.

Your doctor should give you a complete physical exam (you should get a complete physical exam once a year), including:

- measuring your height, weight, pulse, and blood pressure
- checking your legs, feet, hands, fingers, mouth, and eyes
- checking your neck (for possible thyroid problems), feeling your abdomen, and listening to your heart with a stethoscope
- checking your skin, especially where you inject insulin
- testing your reflexes
- conducting the blood and urine tests described below

Your doctor or associated team member should also work with you to design a plan for managing your diabetes. In order to do this she should ask you questions about your dieting and weight habits and your past and current lifestyle, exercise, and eating habits. She should also ask you how often you have had ketones (toxic acid) in your urine and low blood glucose reactions.

She should take into account your personal schedule, including what and when you like to eat, when you like to exercise, and when you work. Your cultural background and food preferences should also be factored into the eating equation.

Finally, she should tell you who you will also need to see (such as an eye or foot specialist) and how often. Before you leave the office make sure you know when your next checkup is. If you take insulin or if you're having problems controlling your glucose levels, you may need to see your doctor at least four times a year (even more often if you are having complications).

Follow-up Visits

You should have at least one member of your health care team closely follow-ing your day-to-day progress. In my experience, this might be a certified diabetes educator. These professionals are often nurses or dietitians who have been specially trained and certified in diabetes management. On follow-up visits they should ask to see your blood glucose records. You should tell them if you have had any problems following your diabetes care plan and if you've made any adjustments to the plan. If you've had any high or low blood glu-cose incidences or symptoms that might relate to possible complications, now would be the time to describe them.

One of the most important parts of the follow-up visit is for the health care team to review your treatment plan and talk about progress or problems in meeting the agreed-upon goals.

On follow-up visits your health care team should be measuring your weight and blood pressure and taking blood for a glycohemoglobin test and urine to test for protein and infection. They should also look at your feet and eyes.

Blood and Urine Tests

You'll be seeing your health care team regularly for testing. One of the two most important tests is glycohemoglobin, which measures your average blood glucose level over the past two to three months. The other important test is for your urine protein level.

Since the incidence of cardiovascular disease is so much greater in people with diabetes, all diabetic adults should be screened for blood lipid levels *more* often than is recommended by the National Cholesterol Education Project Guidelines for healthy adults. Make sure you get a complete workup for tri-glycerides, cholesterol, and high-density lipoprotein (HDL) and low-density lipoprotein (LDL) cholesterol.

Information on Common Medical Treatments

Make sure your health care team goes over the more common medical treat-ments for people with diabetes. You should have some input into which medications (if any) will be part of your personalized diabetes treatment plan, even if that means insisting only on knowing what each medication does, including its side effects.

Considering all the new pharmaceuticals available to treat diabetes, people newly diagnosed with diabetes will find numerous treatment options today that were not available in the recent past. Some medications, such as metformin, Glucophage, or Rezulin, help make certain people more sensitive to the insulin their bodies are already producing. Another drug, Precose (acarbose), delays digestion of carbohydrates and helps prevent some of the carbohydrate you eat from being absorbed. Amaryl helps stimulate insulin production in the pancreas, and Humalog, another new drug, is an ultra-short-acting human-derived insulin. And according to many diabetes specialists, even more helpful diabetes medications are soon to come.

Many pharmaceutical treatments can be successfully used in combination with one another, such as Amaryl with Rezulin, or Glucophage, or insulin with sulfonylureas (oral hypoglycemics that help your pancreas produce more insulin). Your health care team may have to spend time trying out certain treatments, and adjusting the doses, to find a good fit for you.

Insulin.   I appreciate that as someone with diabetes, you're probably weary or wary of the subject of insulin. Consider the following a quick refresher course, useful in dealing with your health care team or in your new role as captain. You're the boss, so you'll want to understand what your expert advisers are saying.

It is odd that someone with Type II diabetes, a condition also called "non–insulin dependent" diabetes, could be "dependent" on insulin. But that's exactly what happens to most Type II diabetics; after ten to fifteen years with the disease, they require insulin for metabolic control. True, at first they may not have been dependent on insulin—because their bodies still produced the hormone. What happened was that their body cells were *resistant* to the insulin. Think of your body's new resistance as changing the lock on the door so that the key (insulin) no longer works.

That's important because insulin is a hormone essential for three vital metabolic systems.

1. *Metabolism of carbohydrates* (the breakdown of carbohydrates into energy). All carbohydrates are eventually broken down into glucose, and glucose needs insulin to be able to enter most body cells. Insulin is the key that opens the door. It also stimulates the body to make glycogen (the storage form of carbohydrate) when there is more glucose around than the body needs. And as glucose enters body cells, insulin helps it convert to triglycerides.

2. *Metabolism of protein* (the breakdown of protein into usable compo-

nents). As insulin lowers blood glucose levels, it also serves to lower blood amino acids (the breakdown product of protein). Insulin assists amino acids in entering tissue protein. It also alters liver enzymes, encouraging glucose to be produced from amino acids when it is needed for energy (gluconeogenesis).

3. *Metabolism of fat.* This is probably the most unpopular job insulin has: Insulin activates the enzyme lipoprotein lipase, which encourages adipose tissue (body fat) to store more triglycerides. To make matters worse, at the same time insulin inhibits the breakdown of body fat for energy (lipolysis) and promotes the production of fat by the liver (hepatic lipogenesis).

But what happens without insulin? The breakdown of fat for energy accelerates. That may sound good to someone wanting to shed extra body fat, but it leads to excessive production of ketones (an acidic end product of fat metabolism), which can eventually result in a very serious condition called diabetic ketoacidosis. Diabetic ketoacidosis is characterized by hyperglycemia (high circulating-blood levels of glucose) and ketosis (high levels of ketone bodies, such as acetone); dehydration; and electrolyte imbalance.

Oral hypoglycemics. Some oral hypoglycemics (also known as sulfonylureas) help your pancreas produce more insulin. Others help the cells to use the insulin your body is still producing more effectively. And some hypoglycemics slow down the rate that your liver produces sugar, thereby lowering your blood glucose. Certain substances, such as alcohol, or medications, such as aspirin, may make your oral hypoglycemic agent more or less effective. Check with your doctor first before using them.

ACE inhibitors. ACE (angiotensin-converting enzyme) inhibitors have been shown to delay the progression of diabetic renal disease in patients with Type II diabetes at almost any stage, even when hypertension is not yet present.

Newer pharmacological treatments to ask about. Metformin is unique because it increases the insulin sensitivity of the body while lowering insulin concentrations (both very desirable outcomes for Type II diabetics). In various U.S. trials it lowered hemoglobin A1c (a measure of how normal the blood sugar has been over time) by about 2 percent compared to the control groups.

Acarbose helps lower blood glucose after meals. It works in the intestinal tract, inhibiting the intestinal enzyme responsible for carbohydrate absorption. Acarbose has been shown to lower hemoglobin A1c between .5 percent and 1 percent without increasing insulin. Friends of mine are using acarbose and report that it has really helped them gain better blood glucose control. However, because it prevents some carbohydrate from being absorbed in the intestines, there are a few potentially embarrassing intestinal side effects, such as gas and soft stools.

Instructions on Monitoring Glucose Levels

Monitoring is one of the keys to successfully managing diabetes. You need to know what your blood sugar is to know if your blood glucose levels are dangerously high or low from day to day. Measuring your blood glucose will also tell you whether you are meeting your treatment goals and whether the agreed-upon treatments (diet, exercise, or pharmacological) are working.

Make sure someone on your health care team clearly demonstrates how to measure your glucose and how to record it so it can be referred to easily at follow-up visits.

Establishing Emergency Procedures

Be very clear with your health care team what justifies an emergency—that is, establish when should you contact them immediately. Often they will want to be called if you've had nausea and vomiting to the point that you can't eat or if you've had a fever for more than a day. Should you call the doctor (or another member of the health care team) when your blood glucose is too high or too low? What number is considered too high and what number is considered too low? If you are making big changes in your diabetes treatment, your doctor or health care team may want you to make regular reports. Write down the phone numbers you will need for office hours, on-call situations, and hospital emergencies.

Individualization for Diet Therapy

No one diet is best for all people with diabetes. Sometimes a lower-fat, higher-carbohydrate diet is more acceptable and other times a lower-carbohydrate diet high in monounsaturated fatty acids (using mostly canola and olive oils and avocado) is better tolerated. It is you (and maybe your significant others) who has to live with the eating plan, probably for the rest of your life. It behooves you and your health care team to consider your lifestyle, food preferences, cultural background, and so on when designing that eating plan.

References for Additional Information and Assistance

A reference sheet including numbers for national diabetes groups and local counselors, support groups, fitness clubs, and dietitians—all specializing in diabetes—can be an indispensable guide to finding the right help at the right time. If your health care team members do not have a reference sheet to offer you for additional help and information, find someone who does. Many hospitals have diabetes support groups, and that's a great place to start.

OTHER MEMBERS OF YOUR HEALTH CARE TEAM

One physician can't possibly be an expert in every aspect of diabetes therapy. Obviously, a pharmacist is going to know more about medications; a dietitian is going to know more about changing eating habits, different foods, and nutrition therapy; a podiatrist is going to know about feet; and the ophthalmologist about eyes. All these professionals are the other members of your health care team, and they are all vital to the success of the team and your diabetes management.

Still other possible teammates that might be needed are an endocrinologist, a certified diabetes educator, a behavioral specialist, a psychologist, and/or a nephrologist, depending on your particular and changing needs. I've already mentioned that having an expert in exercise for people with diabetes can be very useful in establishing a safe program that you might actually enjoy following (one of the keys to success).

You should recruit all of these people the same way you chose—or redefined your relationship with—your personal physician. You should be comfortable working together and exchanging information. You want good teammates, captain.

AND DON'T FORGET YOUR FAMILY

Doctors and specialists of various kinds see you from time to time, but your family is with you every day. You'll need them for support and to help make the lifestyle changes that will lead to better control of your diabetes. Make them part of your team by sharing—as much as you think useful and appropriate—the information in this book and your strategy for managing your condition. If needed, family therapists or counselors should be available to help you and your family and redefine treatment roles.

ONCE AGAIN, THE GOOD NEWS

Family members also get to participate in the upside of your more active involvement in personalized and flexible diabetes management. That is, better and more satisfying dining. I'll get to the real payoff in the final chapter: Recipes You Need and Recipes You Asked For. But first, let's dig in to all the good nutrition information served up in the next three chapters. You'll need to discover just what you can and should be eating.

2

GOOD NEWS FOR THOSE
WHO ENJOY EATING

Whether you've been dealing with diabetes for years or you've just been diagnosed, it's about time you got some good news, isn't it? You probably feel as if your life is a long list of diet don'ts. And you probably spend some of your day beating yourself up over what you "shouldn't" have eaten. Well, the shackles are finally loosening a little. You *can* have sugar (but please note the fine print: "Some rules and restrictions apply"). You might also be one of the many people with diabetes who *can* have a moderate amount of alcohol (again, "some rules and restrictions apply"). Still more good news: carbohydrates are *not the enemy*. In fact, for many people with diabetes a high-carbohydrate diet, also rich in soluble fiber, may be ideal. Oil is *not the enemy* either, particularly oils rich in monounsaturated fat. And never before have those with diabetes had such a wide selection of sugar-free or light products to choose from, using an arsenal of artificial and low-calorie sweeteners. And if that wasn't enough good news—you may not have to lose *all* your extra weight to see an improvement in your diabetes: Indeed, 10 to 20 pounds may be just the ticket to feeling better and to better glucose control.

But first, there is one more important disclaimer: *General recommendations regarding the composition of diabetes diets should be viewed as average values for a whole group of patients with a range of possible variations for individuals with different needs.*

That is why medical and health generalizations are qualified with "most," "many," and "some." You may individualize your treatment with the aid of your team for better control and happier living.

THE BUDDY SYSTEM: PAIRING
CARBOHYDRATES WITH FAT OR PROTEIN

Now that you are have diabetes, it's time to say goodbye to meals or snacks that are *completely* carbohydrate. The days of plain bagels, or a big glass of orange juice, or a big bowl of fruit as a snack are gone forever. But that doesn't sound so bad, does it? A glass of juice usually tastes better when you are washing down your breakfast. How good was a plain bagel anyway? You can still have your bagel; you just need to find a partner that is high in protein or fat to eat with it. How about some light cream cheese or peanut butter on that bagel?

Your body handles carbohydrates better when they are ingested with protein and fat. Yes, it's true; someone is actually telling you that you need fat! Fat helps lower the blood glucose response of the other foods it is eaten with. The bottom line here is *balance*: pairing your high-carbohydrate foods (fruits, breads, starches, beans) with foods that will contribute some protein and fat.

While carbohydrates are completely converted to sugar in the blood for energy, only 50 percent of all protein and just 10 percent of food fat is converted to blood sugar. But before you go guzzling olive oil or slicing into that cube of butter, there is something else you should know. Your calories from fat will add up quickly because each gram of fat contributes at least 9 calories (more than twice the calories a gram of carbohydrate or protein contributes). So you definitely want *some* fat in every meal and snack to balance the carbohydrates—but not too much.

You definitely want some protein in every meal and snack, too. But again, you probably don't want to go overboard. Your body prefers to get the majority of its fuel (energy) from carbohydrates. And most protein foods, particularly animal protein (some more than others), come with their fair share of saturated fat and cholesterol. Last, it's a good idea for most diabetics to avoid excessive amounts of protein to prevent any undue stress on the kidneys, thus possibly delaying any potential complications with those vulnerable and vital organs. Experimental and clinical studies show that protein restriction, as an adjunct to blood pressure control, slows the progression of renal disease by reducing albuminuria and preserving renal function.

Americans get about 12 to 20 percent of their total calories from protein. This is nearly two times the amount actually required by the body. How much protein should people with diabetes be consuming? Unfortunately, we don't know the ideal percentage. However, although we may not know what is ideal, we do know what is required to meet normal protein needs for most adults—1 gram of protein per kilogram of body weight.

I realize that at first glance the information doesn't sound very helpful, but the calculations are not difficult. And once you do them, the modifications for when you lose weight are even easier.

For example, one of my editors conveniently happens to weigh a nice, round 220 pounds. To find his weight in kilograms, we divide by 2.2, because there are 2.2 pounds per kilo. So Ed, as we will call him, weighs 100 kilos and needs 100 grams of protein daily. Because each gram of protein contains 4 calories, Ed should get 400 calories a day from protein. Just how many total calories Ed should consume (and how many from carbohydrates, fat, and protein) would be decided by Ed and his health care team. Chapter 5 details how to calculate those proportions; it's not as intimidating as you might think.

That doesn't mean there are no complications. The figures change, for instance, if you develop microalbuminuria (a small amount of protein in the urine). The protein content of your diet should then be reduced to 0.8 gram of protein per kilogram of body weight per day. Nor is all protein created equal; some comes with less cholesterol and fat than others. My dietitian's intuition says that getting a significant amount of your protein needs met via plant sources (beans, tofu, vegetables, and grains) rather than from animal sources (meat, dairy) may be beneficial toward the preservation of kidney function. However, the matter is currently being researched.

But back to the main point: every recipe in this book, whether a snack or entree, tries to balance carbohydrate with protein and fat. They work better together.

HIGH-CARBOHYDRATE, HIGH-FIBER FOODS— AT EVERY MEAL

Certainly everyone agrees that carbohydrates are important for every meal, but just how much carbohydrate there should be is less certain. This is a hot button for diabetes researchers, particularly where Type II people are concerned. Some say 40 percent of calories should come from carbohydrates, but most contend the figure should be 55 to 60 percent.

Obtaining 60 percent of one's calories from carbohydrates might lead to elevated levels of blood glucose, insulin, and triglycerides after meals. However, recent research has suggested that when a high-carbohydrate diet is also high in fiber (some would say *very* high) these potentially negative health effects are lessened if not eliminated. Therefore, check your blood triglyceride and cholesterol levels during your regular doctor visits to see whether eating high carbohydrates and high fiber is having a persistently positive or negative effect on your blood lipids.

But if we are eating fewer carbohydrates to equal 40 percent of our calories, what should we eat to fill the gap? Some researchers propose mono-unsaturated fat.

For now, the best resolution is to follow the American Diabetes Association recommendations. (See chapter 3 for details.) They emphasize the need to *individualize* the amount of carbohydrate in the meal plan. Your health care team should consider your parameters and current eating habits, as well as the degree of change you are willing to make in your habits and the impact that the type and amount of carbohydrate has on your particular blood glucose and lipid levels.

The Fiber Portion of the Equation

Nutritionists have always given fiber good lip service as a way to prevent constipation (and possibly colon cancer) and as "part of an overall healthy diet." But for those with diabetes, the benefits of water-soluble fiber in particular go way beyond mere prevention. Water-soluble fiber seems to be a vital component of blood glucose control.

Soluble fiber is found in peas and beans, oats and oat bran, barley, and some fruits and vegetables. There are so many benefits to eating a high-fiber diet that, frankly, I don't know where to start. Some research suggests that a diabetes diet obtaining 55 to 60 percent of its calories from complex carbohydrates, less than 30 percent of its calories from fat, and approximately 30 to 40 grams of fiber a day:

• *Improves blood glucose control.* Fiber, especially the water-soluble variety, may slow carbohydrate absorption and lessen the rise in blood glucose and insulin that follows every meal by forming a gel within the intestinal tract.

• *Reduces levels of atherosclerosis-promoting blood lipids.* It appears that soluble fiber helps lessen the potential elevation of plasma triglycerides and serum lipids observed in some diabetics who consume a high-carbohydrate diet.

• *Decreases blood pressure in those with high blood pressure (hypertension).*

• *Reduces body weight in the obese.* The fat we eat is more likely to be stored as body fat than are carbohydrates. A gram of fat also contributes almost twice as many calories as a gram of carbohydrate. Therefore, a high-fat diet is more likely to be high in calories, compared to a high-carbohydrate diet (rich in complex carbohydrates such as fruits, vegetables, and whole grains). So, if weight loss or weight maintenance is a necessity, trying a high-carbohydrate, high-fiber diet first, rather than a high-fat diet, is probably best.

While water-soluble fibers have been shown to lower serum cholesterol levels, it is the insoluble fibers that help increase stool bulk and decrease the transit time of the stool, helping prevent constipation. Both fibers help us feel full faster when they are part of the meal, possibly discouraging overeating.

• *Improves tissue-insulin sensitivity* (thus, may reduce or eliminate insulin requirements in insulin-treated Type II diabetes).

One study with Type II people (*Diabetes Care* 14, no. 12, December 1991) demonstrated that a high-fiber eating plan reduced insulin requirements by 75 percent, and some people were actually able to get off insulin altogether. Apparently this plan is more effective at lowering postmeal glucose levels and glycohemoglobin values than it is at lowering fasting glucose. This distinction matters because diabetics spend more time in the postmeal state than in the fasting state.

These researchers also discovered that fiber may be even more powerful for blood glucose control than previously thought. They found that the fiber eaten at a meal actually has a beneficial effect on glucose tolerance in the meals immediately following. Their study also showed a 24 percent reduction in serum cholesterol. However, the effects this eating plan had on lowering serum triglycerides were more variable.

How much fiber are we talking about? Some scientists recommend an amount that is too much to be realistic: 30 to 40 grams a day. The average fiber intake for women is 13 grams a day and 19 grams for men. That's a large shortfall. Consequently, some diabetes researchers believe 30 to 40 grams of fiber is impractical and we should rethink the suggested high-carbohydrate diet for some diabetics. However, I think otherwise. With the right tips and recipes, and with a newly acquired taste for beans or perhaps the ability to wash down a scoop of a high-soluble-fiber supplement, many people can meet this ideal 30 to 40 grams at least five days out of seven.

Eating large amounts of fiber and beans doesn't come without its share of uninvited side effects and discomforts. The most common side effects are diarrhea, flatulence, bloatedness, and abdominal pain. To minimize these, increase your fiber gradually and don't forget to drink plenty of water. And if you have a particular problem with beans, try Beano, a commercial product you eat along with beans, cabbage, broccoli, and other vegetables. It contains an enzyme that reduces the various side effects. (Beano is available in most pharmacies and drugstores.) For most people, the above symptoms typically subside within a week or so of starting a high-fiber diet; so hang in there!

For specific tips for upping your fiber, see chapter 6.

MONO- VERSUS POLYUNSATURATED FAT

The fight is on. Polyunsaturated fat was the oil with the brightest future when I was in college in the late seventies. Owing to research conducted in the early nineties, however, the torch is now being passed to the monounsaturated fats. We get monounsaturates mainly from four oils—olive, canola, avocado, and peanut. Olive oil is probably the most popular monounsaturated oil, but I've got my money on canola oil for two reasons.

First, canola oil is flavorless and therefore can be used in *all* dishes, including brownie recipes, fried chicken, and so on. Second, it can be used at higher cooking temperatures without breaking down and smoking. Olive oil, because of its distinctive flavor and because it may break down and smoke when heated to higher temperatures, is somewhat confined to cold dishes and pastas. Don't get me wrong, I love olive oil and I use it often. I've actually got both oils in my cabinet—canola oil for baking and most cooking, and olive oil for Italian recipes and salad dressings. If you really want to get fancy, you can add peanut oil to your monounsaturated fat repertoire and use it for Asian dishes and stir-frying.

Monounsaturated fat's rise to fame is directly related to the fall of saturated fat. Over the years research has documented the hazards of a diet rich in saturated fats (actually, saturated fat has a larger impact on blood cholesterol levels than cholesterol in food). And one way to reduce the amount of saturated fat in food is to replace it with monounsaturated fat.

Current conventional dietary wisdom says no more than 10 percent of daily calories should come from saturated fat, and 300 milligrams or less for dietary cholesterol (ideally no more than 200 to 300 milligrams). Further, any additional fat in the diet should be monounsaturated or polyunsaturated. But this last bit of advice may be changing soon. There is quite a bit of convincing evidence that if the percentage of calories from fat is increased, it should be from monounsaturated sources only.

Here are some of the general health advantages for choosing mostly monounsaturated fats as part of anyone's healthy diet:

- Monounsaturated fat lowers total blood cholesterol levels without reducing HDL cholesterol levels. Polyunsaturated fat lowers total cholesterol levels, but it may also lower HDL cholesterol levels.

• Substituting mono- for polyunsaturated fat decreases the likelihood of LDL cholesterol oxidation.* And LDL oxidation is now thought to encourage LDLs to deposit in arterial walls (a precursor to atherosclerosis).

Here are some of the possible health advantages to choosing mostly monounsaturated fats as part of a diabetic diet:

• High-carbohydrate diets tend to increase plasma triglyceride concentrations in people with Type II diabetes. One way around this problem for diabetics with already elevated serum triglycerides is to reduce their carbohydrates and raise the amount of monounsaturated fat. The research is encouraging, though not conclusive.

In two recent studies, Type II people were put on just such a diet (moderate carbohydrate with high monounsaturated fat). They tended to have lower fasting triglyceride levels, lower daylong glucose levels, and lower daylong insulin levels compared to those on a high-carbohydrate and low-fat diet. However, glycohemoglobin levels, one of the best ways to measure diabetic control, were the same on both the low-fat and high-monounsaturated-fat diets in one of the studies.

Total serum cholesterol, LDL, and HDL cholesterol were no different between the high- and moderate-carbohydrate diets in one of the studies. What I find most troubling is that research from two similar studies on Type II people showed no improvement in any of the blood lipid levels in the high-monounsaturated-fat groups—including serum triglycerides.

• At least one study has shown a reduction in daytime systolic and diastolic blood pressure while Type II people were being treated with a diet rich in monounsaturated fat.

Who Should Switch to a
High-Monounsaturated-Fat Diet?

Who should switch to a moderate (40 to 50 percent of calories) carbohydrate and high-monounsaturated-fat diet? A high-carbohydrate diet, by compari-

*Some promising research suggests that LDLs promote the formation of plaque only after undergoing oxidation (exposure to oxygen) by free radicals inside the artery wall.

son, would be around 55 to 60 percent of calories. If you find this question perplexing, you are in good company. The answer to this question is currently being debated by the top diabetes researchers across the globe.

The biggest issue with a high-*carbohydrate* diet is the potential to raise serum triglyceride levels. According to research, this problem eases for the most part when the high-carbohydrate diet is also very high in fiber, particularly soluble fiber (found in oats and barley, beans and peas, apples and citrus fruits).

The biggest issue with a *high-monounsaturated-fat* diet is that it is probably *not* going to encourage the weight loss that many Type II people desperately need. I find it interesting that the studies conducted on the benefits of a high-monounsaturated-fat diet rarely mention any weight changes. (Only one study noted a slight weight loss in both the high-carbohydrate and high-monounsaturated-fat study groups.)

You see, the studies don't report whether the subjects are overweight Type II people. Nor are we told whether these Type II people were in generally poor control or good control of their condition. Most of these studies used Type II people treated with diet alone or oral hypoglycemics. Are these results applicable then to the large portion of Type II people who are in poor control or on insulin?

Many prominent researchers urge caution in prescribing a high-monounsaturated-fat diet as an alternative to high-carbohydrate diets, at least until we know the long-term implications of making such a step. It is possible that a high-fat diet, even when rich in monounsaturated fats, could increase your risk of other diseases, such as cancer.

As you can see, we still have many questions to answer. My best guess is that a high-carbohydrate and low-fat diet (particularly low in saturated fat), with a possible doubling of fiber, is probably best for many Type II people. However, a higher fat (monounsaturated-rich) diet might be considered for (1) Type II diabetics *without* a weight problem, or for those with high triglyceride levels or hypertension, or (2) diabetics who are unable or unwilling to eat about 30 grams of soluble fiber a day as part of their high-carbohydrate diet.

Perhaps the most important questions are "Which type of eating plan would you be more comfortable with?" "Which would you find more enjoyable (and thus be more likely to continue to follow through the years)?" Some people may be more or less culturally comfortable with the high-monounsaturated-fat diet versus the high-fiber and high-carbohydrate diet. Ultimately you need to make this decision with your health care team, weighing all the pros and cons specific to you, your lifestyle, and your medical risk factors.

SUGAR IS NO LONGER TABOO

A "diabetic diet" is no longer synonymous with "sugar-free." Why? New research has shown that sugars and starches affect blood glucose levels similarly. The total amount of food eaten, along with the total amount of carbohydrate, actually has *more* of an effect on blood glucose levels than where the carbohydrate came from. Hip hip hooray! Can you say *sugar*? I knew you could.

For years sugar has been a forbidden pleasure for diabetics. When you were diagnosed with diabetes, "no more sugar" seemed to be the next words out of the doctor's or dietitian's mouth. Common medical wisdom assumed that because sugars are simple carbohydrates, they are absorbed more quickly into the bloodstream and thus would cause a more dramatic increase in blood sugar compared to complex carbohydrates. The truth is that bread and several other starches have almost the same effect on blood sugar that refined sugar does. So the 1994 recommendations from the American Diabetes Association (ADA) now say: If you are managing your blood sugar well, then *yes*, you may have some sugar—but not too much.

You knew there would be a catch, didn't you? If diabetics are going to use sugars and still control their blood sugar, they have to play by the rules. Start by looking closely at this statement from the ADA: "The addition of *moderate amounts of sugar* in the diet, *as part of ordinary meals*, does not impair blood glucose control in diabetics as long as *sucrose is substituted for other carbohydrate-rich foods*." So, now you have four rules to follow:

1. *Pay attention to portion sizes of sugary foods.* One source defined a portion as "5 to 10 grams of sucrose in a meal." If you are eating a dessert-type food that also contains starch, such as a brownie, *ideally* your total carbohydrate (sugar plus flour) might be more in the order of 15 grams, though it should be no more than 30 grams. Be forewarned: we aren't talking about great big servings you can really sink your teeth into. We mean a single serving of a reduced-sugar cocoa brownie (see recipe on page 210), or one-half cup of light ice cream, or three Oreo cookies.

2. *Try to enjoy your dessert or high-sugar snack as part of a meal.* If you don't have your sugar treat as an extra or separate snack, you'll be more likely to eat reasonable (not excessive) amounts. And just as important, the dessert or snack will be less likely to send your blood sugar soaring if it's paired with other foods contributing protein, fiber, and fat.

3. *Substitute the sugar-containing food for another carbohydrate-*

containing food as part of your diabetic meal plan. In other words, don't eat the sugary food as an extra carbohydrate—in addition to the other carbohydrate foods in your meal plan. Otherwise, you will not only increase the carbohydrates you're taking in, you'll also increase your calories.

4. *Monitor your blood glucose routinely so you'll be aware of any negative effects from the sugar.* You're doing this already, as one of the three keys to successfully managing your diabetes. Eternal vigilance is the price of the freedom to eat sugar.

So, let yourself eat cake, but a modest slice—that's really what the new recommendations are telling us. This can be like letting a child loose in a candy store and telling her to pick just one thing. That works with some kids, but it can be very hard for others. Remember rule 3. If you use your carbohydrate allotment on high-sugar foods and desserts, you lose the nutritional value (vitamins, minerals, cancer-fighting phytochemicals, fiber, etc.) of foods like fruits and grains compared to high-sugar foods. I know that this idea probably brings little motivation or comfort when you are face to face with a large piece of rich chocolate cake or a Snickers bar.

Please be aware that you must still be careful of foods that contain high amounts of added sugars, such as regular soft drinks, syrups, rich desserts, and so on. These foods are on your Eater Beware list not only because they contain high amounts of carbohydrate but because they sometimes contain high amounts of calories and fat as well.

Finally, there is some evidence that larger amounts of added sugar may make metabolic control in Type II diabetes more difficult when such use is continued over a longer time. So find the balance between enjoying some of your favorite sugar-containing foods in moderate amounts (rule 1) as part of a healthful meal (rule 2), substituting the total grams of carbohydrate it contributes for other carbohydrates in the meal (rule 3). Make sure these foods are truly satisfying, so you'll be happy with the moderate amounts—and you'll have it made.

HOW SWEET IT IS: THE LATEST ON ALTERNATIVE SWEETENERS

There's a food rule in our house (and we don't have many)—only one can of diet soda a day. This rule exists not only for my two children but for me as well. There are two reasons for this food rule. First, I am leery of feeding large amounts of artificial anything to children. Second, if water is the best beverage for your body, then water is what you should be drinking most of the time. And obviously you are more likely to be drinking water if you're not drinking diet sodas.

Before I started working on this book, my one Diet Pepsi a day was the extent of my artificial sweetener intake. I'm pretty sensitive to the aftertaste of saccharin and the intensity of aspartame, so I avoided yogurts or frozen desserts that used them. But now that I have talked to my share of diabetics, tasted my share of artificially sweetened products, and created a collection of low-sugar recipes, I have a slight appreciation for alternative sweeteners.

I think artificial sweeteners work best when they are used in small amounts and perhaps as supplements to a small amount of real sugar. (I often use saccharin or aspartame in combination with a small amount of sugar in some of the recipes in this book.) I tend not to notice the aftertaste of saccharin or the intensity of aspartame if only small amounts are added.

I've always suspected, given my own experience, that artificial sweeteners somehow increased our appetite or desire for the real thing, that is, for sugar, which is another reason why I try not to consume it regularly in larger quantities. Sure enough, in some research studies saccharin and aspartame increased the hunger for sugar in test subjects.

Other research has found that aspartame-sweetened soft drinks are associated with weight loss in men—but not in women. This is ironic considering women are the ones who drink most of the diet soft drinks in efforts to reduce their weight. Since I am a woman who is constantly battling the bulge, this finding disturbs me.

I can't count the times I've seen people order a diet soda in a restaurant and then also order a big chunk of cake or pie. I've probably also done it myself a time or two. The point is we need to be sure we don't rationalize eating other high-calorie foods simply because we are saving a few calories by drinking a diet soda or eating an artificially sweetened food. Enough said.

Here is a review of the various alternative sweeteners—some natural, some synthetic, some contributing calories, some calorie-free.

Aspartame (NutraSweet, Equal)

What would you say if I told you I had a sweetener that was two hundred times sweeter than sugar, contributes negligible calories, doesn't raise blood glucose levels, and is described as having a "clean-tasting flavor"? Would you say it sounds too good to be true? NutraSweet has all that. Its one weakness is that it loses its sweetness when heated. The only time NutraSweet can be used for baking is when some acid ingredient is present (such as with apple pie). Your only other alternative is to add it at the end of the cooking process, which doesn't exactly work in the case of cookies, brownies, and cakes.

How easy is it to find NutraSweet in your average supermarket? To say that NutraSweet has infiltrated our food supply over the past ten years would be an understatement. It is currently approved for use in more than 150 different product categories totaling 1,500 specific items. This is, in my opinion, a double-edged sword. While it is great that people, particularly those with diabetes, now have so many products to choose from, the amounts that children and adults can potentially be consuming have never been greater. Just add it up: NutraSweet can be used as a tabletop sweetener, it's in soft drinks, powdered drinks, cocoa mixes, juices, shake mixes, chocolate milks, teas and coffees, yogurt and puddings, gelatins and topping mixes, frozen desserts, cereals, fruit spreads, chewing gums, breath mints, diet products, and some bakery items.

A few researchers would also say NutraSweet has another weakness besides its inability to withstand heat. They suggest that even though blood levels of phenylalanine (one of the two amino acids that make up NutraSweet) appear normal after consuming NutraSweetened foods, the brain levels may be increased. These high levels of phenylalanine in the brain, they propose, are not only changing the brain neurochemistry, they may be inhibiting the enzymes that help synthesize brain serotonin and catecholamine (such as norepinephrine)—promoting everything from headaches to seizures in people who are already at risk.

To those who respond that phenylalanine is found naturally in many protein foods, they would explain that in a normal diet, the natural phenylalanine is absorbed in the presence of other large and neutral amino acids, which then compete with it for uptake into the brain, thereby having a much reduced effect on the brain neurochemistry.

Many researchers agree that aspartame does have the potential to act as an antigen and so some people may have allergic reactions to it. The American Dietetic Association believes that there is evidence that indicates long-term consumption of aspartame is safe and is not associated with any adverse health effects. My advice is to avoid excessive amounts of any artificial sweetener, and if you are noticing any side effects or possible allergic reactions to aspartame, contact your doctor.

Acesulfame-K (Sunette, Sweet One)

Acesulfame-K is an organic salt containing carbon, nitrogen, oxygen, hydrogen, sulfur, and potassium atoms. Like NutraSweet, it is two hundred times sweeter than sugar and has no lingering aftertaste (except when used in high concentrations). But this is where the similarity ends. Unlike NutraSweet, acesulfame-K can be heated and used in cooking. Unlike NutraSweet, the body does not metabolize acesulfame-K, so it is excreted from the body metabolically unchanged. No toxic effects have been identified in the 90-some-odd safety studies conducted. However, one consumer activist group begs to differ. The Center for Science in the Public Interest criticized these studies and urged the FDA to rescind its approval—something about rats and tumors. But according to the position statement of the American Dietetic Association on the use of nutritive and nonnutritive sweeteners, a detailed analysis of the tumors showed that they were typical of what could be routinely expected in rats and were reported not to be related to the acesulfame-K.

Saccharin (Sweet'n Low, Sugar Twin)

Saccharin is the artificial sweetener with the slight bitter aftertaste. Some people are more sensitive to this than others. I might be choking a sugar-free saccharin-containing food down saying, "Ugh, this is awful," while someone else thinks it tastes fine. Chances are you know which type of taster you are by now.

Saccharin is the sweetest of all the alternative sweeteners, three hundred times sweeter than sugar. It can also be used in baking and cooking, since it is stable under heat. The good news is it is not metabolized in the human digestive system and is removed rapidly via urine. The bad news is animal research implicated saccharin as a weak bladder carcinogen in second generation male rats when large doses of saccharin were given. But human studies didn't support this association. According to the American Dietetic Association, saccharin at current intake levels is assumed safe for the general public.

The recommended intake of saccharin for children is 500 milligrams per day (thirteen packets of Sweet'n Low) and 1,000 milligrams per day for adults (twenty-five packets of Sweet'n Low).

Sugar Alcohols (Such as Sorbitol, Mannitol, Xylitol)

Sugar alcohols grow on trees. That's right, sugar alcohols are found naturally in berries, apples, plums, and more. Some of the sugar alcohols are only half as sweet as sugar (sorbitol, mannitol); others are just as sweet as sugar (xylitol, maltitol). Because they don't raise blood sugar as high as sugar and they aren't fully absorbed, they actually contribute fewer calories than other carbohydrates.

Sugar alcohols are considered to be very safe, but I must warn you they can cause some inconvenient side effects in diabetics and nondiabetics alike. I found this out firsthand when I was taste-testing lower sugar products for this book. Trust me, you could experience some abdominal gas and diarrhea, courtesy of the sugar alcohols—particularly sorbitol. How much sugar alcohol will send you into this intestinal tailspin depends on how sensitive your gastrointestinal tract tends to be. For most, it might be 30 grams of sorbitol consumed in a single dose. For others, it could very well be just 10 grams. Take it from one with a rather sensitive tract, you can get to 10 grams pretty fast. If a small hard candy contains 3 grams of sorbitol, then you could be 4 candies away from, well, you know.

One summer my rather worried dad called me because he had persistent diarrhea ever since he got back from his vacation in Hawaii. I asked him if there was anything he was drinking or eating that was different from usual. He mentioned he was drinking sugar-free powdered beverage drinks such as sugar-free lemonade by the gallon. I told him that they contain some sugar substitutes that can, in large amounts, cause diarrhea. He stopped drinking so much of the drink (and started drinking more water) and the diarrhea went away.

I've noticed lately that several of the sugar alcohols are added to many light and fat-free products, probably because they add bulk and texture and help the product retain moisture. In this case, the sweet taste is just a bonus. They do not promote cavities, so sugar alcohols make great sweeteners for chewing gum. Sugar alcohols are also used to sweeten candies and cookies.

Low-Calorie Sweeteners Count, Too

Calories from low-calorie sweeteners should be accounted for in your meal plan because in sufficient quantities they can increase blood glucose levels. They will be included in the grams of carbohydrate per serving on the package.

EAT, DRINK, AND BE MERRY?

As luck would have it, not only is alcohol the only macronutrient that does not require insulin to be metabolized, it even augments the action of insulin.

Because alcohol cannot be converted into glucose by the body, once absorbed it can do one of two things: it can be used as an energy source, or it can be (in excessive amounts) converted to fats. Obviously you want to avoid the latter by drinking only in moderation.

In practice, when alcohol is used in moderation (there's that word again) and if diabetes is well controlled, blood glucose levels are usually not affected. But here's the kicker—a "moderate" amount of alcohol for a diabetic is different from what would be considered "moderate drinking" for the general public. A moderate amount of alcohol for a diabetic is described as two servings of an alcoholic beverage enjoyed once or twice a *week*. A serving of alcohol is equivalent to a 1.5-ounce shot of a distilled beverage, 12 ounces of beer (preferably light), or 4 to 5 ounces of wine (preferably dry).

But wait, I'm not through with the drinking rules yet. Alcohol should be enjoyed with a meal. This is because alcohol inhibits the release of glucose from the liver and can cause hypoglycemia when it is consumed without food. This is not to be taken lightly; the hypoglycemic effect may persist from eight to twelve hours after the last drink. I repeat: food should *not* be omitted because of the possibility of alcohol-induced hypoglycemia. But if alcohol is consumed nearly every day, the calories should be included in the meal plan.

There are a few reasons a Type II diabetic should try to keep alcohol a once- or twice-a-week pleasure at the most. First of all, alcohol is high in calories (7 calories per gram) and is metabolized like fat. In addition, alcohol may interfere with the action of other medications that are being taken (you should check with your doctor before consuming alcohol). Finally, alcohol may raise triglyceride levels. Given that diabetics are at increased risk for coronary artery disease, regular consumption is probably not a great idea. Consider nonalcoholic beers and beverages. Although they still contain some calories and carbohydrates, they are virtually alcohol-free. There are some great-tasting nonalcoholic beers (imported and domestic), and the nonalcoholic wines have come a long way (try Ariel's Zinfandel, Merlot, and Cabernet).

TEN TO TWENTY POUNDS MAY BE ALL YOU HAVE TO LOSE

"Just lose weight" are usually words spoken from the mouths of people who have never had a weight problem. If they truly did have one, they wouldn't say "just." They would understand how difficult it is for some people, through no fault of their own, to shed those extra pounds.

If it's any consolation, and I hope it is, the diabetes experts have eased off their insistence that you lose *all* your extra weight and reduced their recommendation to losing 10 to 20 pounds. You may consider losing 10 to 20 pounds as "just the tip of the iceberg," but that may be enough to improve your blood glucose control. And that may also be enough to improve your confidence and your energy level.

Losing all your extra weight is pie in the sky for most people—destined to end in feelings of failure and possibly depression. Strict dieting gives new meaning to the phrase, "no pain, no gain." If losing the weight is so painful that you constantly feel hungry and deprived, you are destined to gain it all back later—and then some. Instead, losing a more reasonable amount of weight offers you feelings of personal power and success. The most successful type of weight loss is not painful; the changes may be less drastic, but they are more likely to be permanent.

Losing 10 to 20 pounds is not only an attainable goal, it can be enough to turn your boat around in this stormy sea called diabetes. It can get things going in a more healthful direction—healthful for your body and healthful for your psyche.

To find out more about monounsaturated fats; losing weight, slow but sure; and balancing carbohydrates and the best-tasting no-sugar or less-sugar products, stay tuned.

3

NEW DIET GUIDELINES
FROM THE AMERICAN
DIABETES ASSOCIATION

In 1994 history was made. The American Diabetes Association released revolutionary recommendations that would change the way diabetics look at food and the way health professionals look at diabetics, possibly forever. I know that sounds rather dramatic, but the new 1994 recommendations do boldly go where no diabetic diet recommendations have gone before. Many changes were made, some practical, some philosophical, but all very positive for diabetics.

TWO GREAT REASONS TO EAT WELL

There are two reasons to follow your personally designed eating plan closely: (1) to feel better right now, and (2) to feel better years from now.

To Feel Better Now

When your blood sugar is within normal range you feel better. You feel as though you have more energy. Perhaps you are less irritable. You don't have to run to the bathroom as often during the day or interrupt your night's sleep. And when you test your blood sugar and see that it has fallen into the normal range—you've got to feel great about that! That's about as close to instant gratification as you're going to get with diabetes, because the biggest rewards for controlling your blood sugar and lowering blood lipids come down the road.

To Feel Better Later

You know that how you eat today can help prevent or promote various diseases and diabetic complications further down the line. You've been told repeatedly that chronic high blood sugar eventually damages your entire body—the nerves, blood vessels, eyes, heart, kidneys, and other organs. Consequently, if you can reduce your blood sugar to within normal ranges, you will help prevent these complications from happening; you will be more likely to have your nerves, blood vessels, eyes, heart, and kidneys intact in the future. This is the ultimate delayed gratification from all that hard work you are doing to lower your blood sugar now. The same goes for lowering your blood lipids and blood pressure. The true rewards are realized years after you have changed your eating plan and lifestyle.

GENERAL RECOMMENDATIONS AND NEW PERSPECTIVES

Ramifications of the Diabetes Control and Complications Trial

The largest study on people with diabetes ever conducted, the Diabetes Control and Complications Trial (DCCT), involved 1,441 Type I diabetics, aged thirteen to thirty-nine. They were randomly assigned to either conventional or intensive diabetes treatment groups and then followed for three to nine years.

The trial told us a few things. First, that intensive therapy (tight control) can lead to improved blood glucose levels. And second, that improved blood glucose levels can lead to an impressive decrease in long-term diabetes complications. The tight control group reduced their risk of retinopathy (disorder of the retina) up to 76 percent, their risk of nephropathy (disease of the kidney) up to 56 percent, and their risk of neuropathy (disease of the nerves) up to 60 percent.

Because intensive therapy involves *intensive self-monitoring and self-care*, the trial also demonstrated how important it was for *those with diabetes to have more responsibility for their own therapy* by becoming involved *members of the team*. And finally, the trial showed that this *individualization of treatment plans and instruction* to ensure successful diabetes self-management takes time; many hours of interaction between the diabetic and the health care team were needed in the intensive treatment group.

Is Blood Sugar Control for Type II, Too?

I know what you're thinking—"This trial doesn't relate to me; I have Type II diabetes." Although the DCCT included only Type I people, many experts have commented that there is *no* reason not to believe that tight glucose control would also benefit Type IIs. In fact, that is the ADA's thinking.

A six-year study was recently completed on Japanese Type II people, demonstrating that tight blood glucose control is effective in delaying the onset and progression of microvascular (small blood vessel) complications. But just how well these results transfer to the American Type II population is still debatable. You see, the Japanese Type IIs were not only lean, but also had normal blood pressure and blood lipid levels. American Type II diabetics, on the other hand, tend to be overweight, and many also battle high blood pressure and elevated blood lipids.

But still, Type II people have one very important thing in common with the people who participated in these two intensive treatment trials. Type IIs are also at risk for the common complications of diabetes. And both trials proved that blood sugar levels directly affect the development of complications.

You can also test your blood sugar more often, as people in the trials did, to get a better picture of how well your blood sugar is being controlled. For example, your health care team may suggest you test your blood sugar before breakfast and either before dinner or before going to bed.

Intensive Insulin Therapy

If diet, exercise, oral agents, and conventional insulin therapy don't get your blood glucose levels down to where they need to be, you may want to discuss intensive insulin therapy with your health care team— this is a frequent insulin routine similar to what people with Type I were practicing in the trial described above. But intensive insulin therapy is not for everyone. Elderly people, for example, or people with heart disease should not use intensive insulin therapy. If you do try intensive insulin therapy, continue to do the other things that will also help you get tight control of your blood sugar, such as eating a healthy diet, losing some excess weight, and exercising.

I've always said that behind every silver lining is a gray cloud. There appears to be a downside to the intensive therapy practiced in the DCCT. The tighter control group had a three times higher incidence of hypoglycemia, that is, abnormally low blood sugar. This condition can be life-threatening for older people and people with cardiovascular disease because it can lead to stroke or heart attack. They also experienced some weight gain. The risk of becoming overweight was 73 percent higher in the intensive therapy group than with conventional therapy.

Of course, this trial was conducted on Type I people (not Type II), but I think we can still learn from the findings, both the positive and the negative. The increased risk of hypoglycemia is probably not as much of a concern for Type II people as is the increased risk of weight gain. That development could pose a difficult choice for the majority of Type IIs who are trying to *lower* (not raise) their weight.

Philosophically Speaking

The American Diabetic Association diet recommendations reflect a new perspective. The new "intensive therapy" embraces a major shift in thinking. A rigid and restrictive set of diet guidelines is now "out," while individualization and flexibility are "in." And instead of the doctor dictating the treatment plan to the patient, treatment is a collaboration between the patient and the health care team. Now doesn't that sound better?

For the first time in almost seventy-five years the American Diabetes Association has rejected the idea of promoting the same proportion of major nutrients for everyone in favor of recommending a diet of 10 to 20 percent of calories from protein and less than 10 percent of calories from saturated fat. Instead, your meal plan must be based on *your* individual medical needs and lifestyle (preferably developed with expert assistance from a registered dietitian and/or certified diabetes educator).

Specifically, you and your team may want to consider any of the following issues when formulating your diet plan:

- What are your day-to-day blood sugars like?
- Are you overweight?
- Have you already tried to reduce your weight a little with a low-fat eating plan that includes exercise? If so, is it working?
- Are you producing any insulin at all?
- Do you have elevated serum triglycerides or other blood lipids?
- Do you have high blood pressure?
- How old are you?

- How motivated are you to make changes in your eating habits and lifestyle?
- What are your food likes and dislikes? Is there a cultural influence in your eating style?

If you are overweight, a low-fat diet is more likely to help you shed some extra pounds. But if you have already tried it and have been unsuccessful, or if you have severely high serum triglycerides, you might want to discuss the option of raising your monounsaturated fats and lowering your carbohydrates with your health care team.

The individual variations are numerous. The ADA recognizes that your physical and emotional well-being depend on an eating plan that is flexible and personal. But, they don't leave you on your own; the ADA has some useful guidelines for everyone to follow.

HOW MUCH IS RIGHT FOR *MOST*

I know I said no *one* meal plan approach, but you need a place from which to start making your personal adjustments. General recommendations can be made for various nutrients such as protein, saturated fat, cholesterol, fiber, and so forth that will probably benefit most diabetics.

Fat and Saturated Fat

Less fat in your food means less fat on your body. Sounds simple, doesn't it? It isn't—as you probably already know. But it is true that a lifestyle low in fat and high in exercise is probably your best bet if weight loss is your aim. One study fed overweight Type II people food that provided 20 percent of calories from fat and fewer calories overall. And what do you think happened? After sixteen weeks, they lost more weight than the group that was given just a low-calorie diet.

Even if you don't consciously lower your calories but you eat low-fat food, you may *still* notice some weight coming off. In one recent study women who ate around 22 percent of their calories from fat, not attempting to lose weight or eat fewer calories, lost an average of 6.6 pounds after a year.

Most Type II people would probably benefit from losing 10 to 20 pounds, and a low-fat diet is an efficient way to cut calories and extra weight. But if a low-fat eating plan isn't working for you, it might be better to lower carbohydrates a bit and replace them with monounsaturated fat, especially if you have elevated serum triglycerides. This type of eating plan usually emphasizes canola and olive oil, nuts, and avocado. Keep in mind, however, that a high-fat diet contributes to obesity—independent of how many calories are eaten.

The 1994 recommendations not only have to consider potential weight loss benefits of a food plan but also the plan's effect on blood glucose and serum lipids. The recommendations leave room for individual variation in percent of calories from fat—the target amount being dependent on the desired glucose, lipids, and weight loss goals for each particular person. For example, if someone has normal lipid levels and isn't overweight, 30 percent of calories from fat might work well. However, if lowering LDL cholesterol is your primary goal, you might want to aim for a diet with less than 30 percent of calories from fat, less than 7 percent of calories from saturated fat, and less than 200 milligrams of cholesterol.

The 1994 recommendations suggest more exact amounts of two of the three *types* of fats: polyunsaturated and saturated fat. The recommendations are that for most diabetics up to 10 percent of calories should come from polyunsaturated fats and less than 10 percent from saturated fat. So it is really only monounsaturated fat that is truly left to individual variation.

Cholesterol

No matter how high or low the total amount of fat in your diet, saturated fat and cholesterol will always need to be low. The 1994 recommendations state that dietary cholesterol should be limited to 300 milligrams or less. The ADA takes a hard line with saturated fat and cholesterol in an effort to reduce the risk of heart disease. Remember, even if you do not have high serum cholesterol, just having diabetes raises your risk for heart disease.

Carbohydrates and Sugar

The 1994 recommendations focus on the *total amount* of carbohydrate rather than the *type* of carbohydrate. This means that sugar can finally come out of the closet. (I discussed in detail the new rules for sugar consumption in chapter 2.)

For years, scientists have thought that sugars and simple carbohydrates were broken into glucose molecules much faster than starches and other complex carbohydrates, raising blood sugar higher and faster. But recent research has shown us that, like most sugars, starchy complex carbohydrates are broken down into glucose during digestion—raising blood sugars. This means starches such as bread, potatoes, and rice are just as likely as plain white table sugar to provoke a surge in your blood sugar.

The new recommendations, encouraging tighter control of blood sugar, promote a closer accounting of *all* carbohydrate. For some this might mean matching their insulin doses closely with a certain number of carbohydrate grams. For others this might mean making sure not to eat more than a certain number of carbohydrate servings at one time—and spreading them out over the day.

While the battle rages on among scientists about whether a high-carbohydrate or moderately low-carbohydrate diet benefits most Type II people, the new ADA recommendations diplomatically refrain from choosing sides. They state that the percent of calories from carbohydrate should be based on the individual's eating habits and glucose and lipid goals.

The 1994 recommendations do not necessarily offer a proposed cap on intake of sugar or sugar-containing foods. They do state, however, that these foods should be substituted for other carbohydrates and not simply added to the meal. Considering the restrictions put on sugar in past diabetes diet guidelines, I can live with this!

Fiber

You need just as much fiber as someone without diabetes—at least 25 grams and striving for 30 to 40, from a wide variety of foods. According to the 1994 recommendations, getting enough fiber to help lower postmeal blood sugar or blood lipid levels is difficult without using fiber supplements. Apparently we need to eat three times the amount of fiber the average American is eating (8 grams for women and 10 grams for men) and primarily water-soluble fiber (oats, apples and citrus, beans and barley) in order to see benefits for diabetes.

But the recommendations also say we could *all* benefit (people with diabetes and people without it) from at least doubling our fiber. Certainly eating high-fiber foods, in general, would benefit the entire family, and working in some delicious high-soluble-fiber foods such as beans and recipes using oats and oat bran is worth a try. Many people with diabetes may even want to consider supplementing their daily diet with a soluble fiber supplement, perhaps before lipid-lowering medications are prescribed.

Sodium

The chief medical reason to reduce sodium is to help reduce blood pressure. But some people are more sensitive to sodium in food than others, and right now we have no way of knowing who is and who isn't. So the 1994 recommendations reflect sodium guidelines given to the public at large—less than 3,000 milligrams of sodium per day. For people with mild to moderate high blood pressure, 2,400 milligrams or less per day of sodium is recommended.

Alcohol

When diabetes is well controlled, blood glucose levels are not normally affected by moderate amounts of alcohol. What is a moderate amount of alcohol? For people using insulin, two or fewer alcoholic beverages (one alcoholic beverage equals one 12-ounce beer, 5 ounces of wine, or $1^1/2$ ounces distilled spirits) may be drunk as part of the usual eating plan (preferably with a meal). People with a history of alcohol abuse should abstain entirely. And people with diabetes with other medical complications such as pancreatitis, abnormal blood lipids, or neuropathy should consider reduction or abstention from alcohol.

Protein

Extra protein causes extra work for your kidneys. Kidney disease can become a problem after many years of diabetes. Protein restriction together with blood pressure control has been shown to slow the progression of renal disease and to preserve renal function.

Also consider this—vegetable protein may be easier on your kidneys. Vegetable proteins also happen to be lower in fat and saturated fat (benefiting your heart disease prevention and weight loss goals as well). Experts are still investigating whether vegetable proteins have a different effect on renal function from animal proteins and whether there is some benefit to restricting dietary protein before kidney disease sets in.

Whatever the source, your body needs *some* protein to make muscles, bones, skin, hormones, enzymes, antibodies, and other important substances. How much is "some"? The new American Diabetes Association recommendations suggest 10 to 20 percent of calories from protein. When nephropathy (kidney disease) is evident, getting no more than 10 percent of calories from protein is recommended.

Ten to 20 percent of calories from protein on an 1,800-calorie-a-day eating plan computes to 45 to 90 grams of protein. To give you an idea of how this translates into food, here is a list of common protein sources:

- Meat, poultry, fish, and cheese have about 7 grams of protein per ounce (a 3-ounce portion would contain around 21 grams)
- Milk and yogurt have about 8 grams of protein per cup
- Peanut butter contains about 8 grams of protein per 2 tablespoons
- Beans, peas, and lentils have about 7 grams of protein per $1/2$ cup cooked
- Tofu has about 8 grams of protein per $1/2$ cup
- Starches and vegetables have about 2 to 3 grams protein per serving (1 slice or $1/2$ cup)

Eat a chicken breast (21 grams of protein), eat a cup of low-fat yogurt (8 grams of protein), and eat a few servings each of vegetables (9 grams of protein) and starches (9 grams of protein)—and call it a day. You've reached the 10 percent of calories from protein target.

4

NUTRITION GOALS AND STRATEGIES

There are two major nutrition goals in managing Type II diabetes: the first is *good blood glucose control*—that is, achieving and maintaining near-normal blood glucose levels; the second is *achieving and maintaining normal blood lipid levels*. You can reach these goals, as I have suggested, through diet, exercise, and monitoring. You can meet these goals by applying four interlocking strategies and making one attitude adjustment. Granted, these strategies and attitude adjustment are easier said than done. But they are worth looking at, because the payoff is tremendous.

Specifically, most people with Type II diabetes will want to:

1. achieve a *moderate* weight loss
2. make a *moderate* reduction in calorie consumption
3. increase their activity level with an effective and *enjoyable* exercise program
4. space out their meals and avoid large caloric intakes late in the day and evening

Finally, all of these strategies work if you adopt them as long-term lifestyle solutions. Your attitude has to be that you're making reasonable and attainable changes necessary to saving, and even improving, your life. So, go with gladness.

But first, some medical and nutritional background. You don't need to memorize all this information, but you should know enough to have perspective on the strategies for controlling your diabetes and to be able to talk with your health care team.

GOAL #1   CONTROLLING BLOOD GLUCOSE LEVELS

Blood Glucose 101

We've talked a lot about the importance of controlling your blood glucose level, and yet you may not understand how the food you eat becomes part of the blood glucose number you read with the prick of your finger.

Let's start at the beginning. When food is swallowed it travels into the stomach (which has about a 4-cup capacity), where it gets hit with acid and an enzyme that begins to break down protein into smaller particles. If the mouth and stomach absorb anything, it is mostly some glucose found in food.

A meal usually leaves the stomach within 2 to 3 hours after it is eaten. Generally solids take longer than liquids to leave the stomach, and fatty meals take longer than a meal of mostly protein or carbohydrate. The next destination is the small intestine, where nutrients are extracted from food and funneled into the bloodstream. This is when much of your digested food has its first major effect on the blood glucose levels.

Digestion and absorption take place with help from the intestinal wall, gallbladder (which donates bile), and pancreas (which donates digestive enzymes). The food particles are in the small intestine for 3 to 10 hours, depending on whether they are carbohydrate, protein, or fat.

Whatever is left (such as plant fibers, food remnants, and other wastes) continues on to the large intestine, where mostly some minerals and water are absorbed into the intestinal wall. It can be 24 to 72 hours before the remaining waste is eliminated (I trust I don't need to elaborate on this point).

The body must maintain a fairly constant level of glucose in the bloodstream to supply energy for red blood cells and nervous tissue. At rest, the brain, for example, uses 35 percent of the body's energy requirements, mostly from glucose in the bloodstream. If you don't eat enough carbohydrate to supply this glucose, your liver (and kidneys to a lesser extent) will be forced to make glucose from amino acids (protein building blocks). Over time this can compromise your valuable muscle tissue.

Factors That Affect Carbohydrate Absorption and the Glycemic Index

The above description of how food is digested and absorbed is the simplified version. It's more complicated when you start discussing the many factors that influence how well and how fast carbohydrate is digested and absorbed by your body. We know that there is a drastic difference in how various carbohydrate-containing foods affect blood glucose responses when tested under standard conditions in people with and without diabetes. Some of these responses might surprise you. For example, regardless of whether bread is made from whole wheat flour or white flour, it raises the blood sugar almost as high as straight glucose.

The easiest way to discuss the effect that a particular food has on the blood sugar response after it is eaten is to introduce the term *glycemic index*. The glycemic index is a way of expressing the rise of blood glucose after eating a particular food against a standard blood glucose curve after glucose is eaten by the same person.

The glycemic index is usually a number between 25 and 100 (100 being the index for pure glucose and 25 being the index for whole barley). Generally, the lower the number, the lower the blood sugar and insulin response to that food. Typically, a group of about ten people is tested (because of individual variability) with the food, and the glycemic index is the mean, or average, response for the group.

Why do all these carbohydrate-containing foods have such different glycemic indexes? Even the major dietary sugars have very different glycemic indexes (figures are approximate):

glucose	100	
lactose	90	(the natural sugar found in milk and milk products)
honey	75	
sucrose	60	(table sugar)
fructose	20	(the natural sugar found in fruit)

The differences occur because the glycemic index of a food (the blood sugar response to that food) is affected by many factors. Here are most of them:

- The physical form of carbohydrate-containing foods (milling and grinding grains, for example, breaks cell walls and so they are digested and absorbed more quickly)
- Cooking and processing (parboiled rice, for example, has a lower glycemic index than the sticky rice found in Chinese restaurants). When starch is gelatinized with water (as is the case with pasta), it tends to be absorbed more slowly.
- Whether the food also contains fat (reduces the glycemic index, probably because of delayed stomach emptying)

- Whether the food also contains soluble fiber (reduces the postmeal blood sugar response)
- The type of sugar or starch the food contains (amylopectin starch is digested more rapidly than amylose, and the higher the proportion of fructose to glucose in a food, the slower the absorption of the carbohydrate). Barley and legumes have a low glycemic index partly because of the high amounts of soluble fiber and resistant starch they contain.

Even various fruits have drastically different glycemic indexes. Bananas, for example, have one of the highest glycemic indexes of the fruits (53). This phenomenon can be explained, in part, by different amounts of fructose and soluble fiber in fruit. But what will probably shock most people is that many of the fruits (apples—39, oranges—43, grapes—43) actually have *lower* glycemic indexes than certain starches such as potatoes (baked—85), rice (70), and white or whole-grain bread (70). Removing the fiber from bread, rice, or pasta appears to have little effect on the glycemic index. This is good news for white bread and white rice lovers. Soluble fibers, though, like the pectin in fruits and vegetables and the guar and beta-glucan fiber found in beans and oats, have a very powerful effect on lowering the blood glucose response.

Chapter 6 contains an extensive listing of the glycemic indexes for a wide variety of foods.

The Future Is Bright for the Glycemic Index

Technically, the glycemic index tells us only about the effect a food has on blood sugar levels. It doesn't tell us directly about the insulin response to that food. This limitation is one of the biggest criticisms for using glycemic indexes. But in general, researchers have found that insulin responses have followed a listing similar to the glycemic responses. In other words, if the glycemic index for a food is low, the insulin response will probably also be low.

The other criticism of the glycemic index is that it isn't practical because it predicts the blood glucose response to a single food, not mixed meals. But many researchers have found that the glycemic index and insulin indexes of many mixed meals could be predicted very well from the glycemic indexes of their component carbohydrates.

So, given that the major criticisms of the glycemic index may well be on their way to being dismissed, the key question becomes, Can a low glycemic-index eating plan lead to significant changes in blood glucose control in people with diabetes? My dietitian training and instincts tell me that the answer to this question is yes. I have included tables, tips, and recipes in this book highlighting the lower glycemic index carbohydrates (see chapter 6). But because I don't want you to have only my perspective, let me tell you what we know so far about the positive effects of a low glycemic-index diet (most of which includes ample oat bran, pasta, and beans).

Recently there was a twelve-week trial of low and high glycemic-index foods in sixteen Type II people (ten using oral hypoglycemic medication, six treated by diet alone). The low glycemic-index diet (emphasizing pasta, oats, barley, legumes, and rye bread) demonstrated less glucose in urine and lower glycosylated hemoglobin levels. Both diets contained the same total amount of fiber (26 grams). Mind you, this is only the first long-term trial of its kind, but the results are very encouraging!

People with Type II diabetes not on insulin can enjoy the potential glucose-lowering effects of a low glycemic-index diet without worrying about adjusting insulin dosages. But even Type II people on insulin could derive some benefits from eating low glycemic-index foods. One study testing the effect of low glycemic-index foods on Type I children reported reduced insulin needs and lower glycosylated albumin levels (albumin turns over more rapidly than hemoglobin). So perhaps a little insulin goes a longer way?

Higher Satiety and Less Aging on Low Glycemic-Index Foods

I just love it when there are more than a couple of good reasons to eat a certain way. For example, we know of many different reasons to eat more fruits and vegetables: they help prevent certain cancers, they help reduce your risk of heart disease, they increase the amount of fiber in your diet, and on and on. A similarly long list exists for a low glycemic-index eating plan.

Controlled trials have shown that a diet with a low glycemic index improves blood glucose control and lipid levels in patients with diabetes (that's Goals 1 *and* 2). In one analysis considering eleven glycemic-index studies in free-living individuals, modest changes in diets showed a 9 percent reduction in glycosylated hemoglobin and a 16 percent reduction in day-long blood glucose. In another study on people with Type II diabetes, fasting blood glucose went down by 30 percent. As far as Goal 2 goes, this analysis showed a 6 percent average reduction in serum cholesterol, and triglycerides were reduced an average of 9 percent (those with more elevated triglycerides had bigger reductions, of about 20 percent).

What I find really encouraging is that the studies found those with diabetes *not* exercising good control (that is, who typically had higher fasting blood sugars, hyperlipidemia, and were overweight) had even more impressive improvements in blood glucose and lipids, which sounds good to me, and things get even better.

Several studies have shown that the higher the fullness rating (satiety) of a particular food, the lower the glycemic index tends to be. Hunger is less likely to return as soon if you had some low glycemic-index foods in your last meal. This can come in handy if you are trying to eat a little less in order to shed a few pounds. I call this the bean burrito effect. When I was pregnant I noticed that if I had a bean burrito for lunch I wouldn't be hungry until dinnertime. But if I had a sandwich or something similar, I would be ravenous by midafternoon.

It is too soon to tell, but there may be an even better reason to emphasize low glycemic-index foods in diets for those with diabetes and those without. One researcher has speculated that one of the processes that contributes to aging is glycosylation of major body proteins (hemoglobin, albumin, collagen, brain protein, muscle protein, etc.). Remember the small trials of low glycemic-index foods in Type I children mentioned earlier that showed a reduction in glycosylated albumin, and the first large trial on low glycemic-index diets in Type II people that demonstrated lower glycosylated hemoglobin levels? This could be the start of something big.

Common Complications—An Incentive to Control Blood Sugar

Kidney failure, blindness, loss of feeling in your feet, chronic nausea, or diarrhea are enough to send intense fear into anyone. Unfortunately, these are only a few of the many possible complications resulting from Type II diabetes.

I'm not reminding you of these possibilities to make you afraid; fear isn't productive. Turn your fear into power. Be prepared. Put up the barriers to block your attacker. There is a big difference between waiting for an intruder to strike, unprepared in a dark corner of your house with your eyes closed, and being ready for an intruder by locking all your doors, setting an alarm, and having your defense plan ready.

Your best defense when it comes to preventing, postponing, or reducing the severity of common complications is by controlling your blood glucose levels. Many studies have established this relationship again and again. People with the highest glycohemoglobin levels usually have nearly three times the risk of developing retinopathy after ten years. And the risk of the retinopathy progressing was higher in the people with the highest glycohemoglobin levels. Incidentally, the cases that do progress can be treated when detected and treated early enough; so don't miss those ophthalmologist's appointments.

Keeping tight control of your blood glucose levels in order to avoid diabetic retinopathy may also help reduce the risk of stroke. A recent study found that people with retinopathy had a three to four times greater risk of stroke than those who did not have retinopathy, even after considering other stroke risk factors (age, smoking status, gender). The researchers suggest retinopathy and stroke may be closely connected because the small blood vessel damage causing retinopathy in the eyes also takes place at the same time in the small arteries going to the brain.

About 20 percent of Type II people develop nephropathy (kidney damage) that can lead to kidney failure (the percentage increases to 30 to 40 percent of people with Type I diabetes). Again, no matter which complication is in question—high blood pressure, heart disease, kidney disease, eye problems, or nerve damage—controlling your blood glucose levels can help prevent them. The table below illustrates this point. The check marks show what you can control to help prevent each complication.

Table of Complications

Things you can control	High blood pressure	Heart disease	Kidney disease	Eye problems	Nerve damage
	Complications				
Blood glucose	✓	✓	✓	✓	✓
Weight	✓	✓			
Saturated fat		✓			
Sugar					
Protein	✓		✓		
Sodium (salt)	✓	✓	✓		
Alcohol		✓			✓
Medicine	✓	✓	✓	✓	✓
Exercise	✓	✓			
Smoking tobacco	✓	✓			✓

Source: 1995, American Diabetes Association, The American Dietetic Association, "Single-Topic Diabetes Resources." Used with permission.

GOAL #2 NORMALIZING BLOOD LIPID LEVELS

The main reason to normalize blood lipid (fat) levels is to reduce the risk of heart disease. This goal is more important to people with diabetes than you might think—75 percent of people with diabetes die of cardiovascular problems. When you are diagnosed with diabetes you automatically receive one more risk factor for coronary artery disease and cerebrovascular disease. In fact, the prevalence of cardiovascular disease in people with diabetes is two to four times that in the diabetes-free general population—even in the absence of other risk factors such as hypertension, smoking, and lipid abnormalities.

In general, people with diabetes have approximately double the risk of stroke. Some researchers suspect that high blood glucose levels increase the risk of stroke by changing blood lipoproteins and accelerating their oxidation, making them more likely to accumulate in arterial walls leading to the brain. High blood glucose may also, in and of itself, exacerbate the development of blood clots. That's the bad news. Okay, that's the *really* bad news.

Given these circumstances, as a Type II person with diabetes, you must pay even more attention than an American with normal health to factors that can reduce your risk of coronary heart disease and stroke. The good news is there are lifestyle changes you can make to minimize your risk of heart disease and stroke and ways that you can measure your progress (that is, keeping track of glycohemoglobin, low density lipoprotein cholesterol, serum triglycerides, serum cholesterol, blood pressure, and so on).

What are those lifestyle changes specifically recommended for lowering blood cholesterol and blood pressure? They are the same ones used to control blood glucose levels—a low-fat, high-carbohydrate, high-fiber diet (for most people), weight loss, and exercise. Which brings us back to our two nutrition goals, controlling blood glucose and normalizing blood lipids. Here are several things you can do to reach Goal 2.

Know Your Blood Lipid Levels

Keep track of your blood lipid levels. If your doctor hasn't told you what your most recent serum cholesterol, LDL cholesterol, serum triglycerides, or HDL cholesterol values are—ask her. Write the numbers down and track them over time so you know whether they are going up or down and whether they are considered high, borderline high, or normal.

The National Cholesterol Education Program for Adults lipid classification values are as follows:

Cholesterol Levels
Desirable: 200 mg/dl or lower
Borderline high: 200–239 mg/dl
High risk: >240 mg/dl and above

LDL-Cholesterol Levels
Desirable: 130 mg/dl or lower
Borderline high: 130–159 mg/dl
High risk: 160 mg/dl and above

Recommended Triglyceride Levels
Adults: 150 mg/dl or lower

The most common lipid abnormalities in people with Type II diabetes are elevated triglycerides, elevated VLDL (very low-density lipoproteins), and decreased HDL (high-density lipoproteins), or "good" cholesterol.

Many of the dietary approaches that aim to decrease undesirably high lipid levels and to increase undesirably low HDL levels are the same diet approaches suggested to reduce the risk of macrovascular disease (hardening of the arteries and risk of stroke) in people with diabetes—promoting, for the most part, a diet rich in fruits, vegetables, whole grains, and beans, and lower in fat.

Know the Rap: Less Saturated Fat Is Where It's At

Eating less fat overall is a good idea for many people with Type II diabetes, and Americans in general, because the total fat content of a meal can lead to an increase in atherogenic particles in the circulation. A low-fat diet will also encourage body fat loss much better than a high-fat diet. But the emphasis these days, especially when it comes to lowering blood lipids and reducing the risk of heart disease, is to *eat less saturated fat*.

A recent study calculated that if, starting today, Americans reduced their saturated fat intake from 12 percent of calories to 9 percent, about 100,000 first-time coronary events (such as heart attacks) could be prevented by the year 2005.

High amounts of saturated fat in our diet are obviously associated with heart disease. More specifically, saturated fat has been shown to raise the level of bad cholesterol and triglycerides in the blood.

Saturated fat is found in animal fats such as butter, high-fat meat, lard, bacon, whole milk, and whole milk cheeses; in coconut and palm oil; and when vegetable oils are "hydrogenated," as is the case with stick margarine and shortening. Many of the packaged foods we buy (such as crackers, cookies, snack foods, frozen fried foods, pastries, etc.) contain hydrogenated oils. Many of our favorite desserts are also very high in saturated fat.

Make Monounsaturated Fats a Larger Portion of the Total Fat

Monounsaturated fats lower the total serum cholesterol levels. But unlike polyunsaturated fats, they do not lower HDL cholesterol at the same time. You can find monounsaturated fat in olive, peanut, and canola oil, in olives, and in nuts (except walnuts).

Eat More Fish

All of us would probably benefit from eating more fish, especially those high in omega-3 fatty acids. Fish oils have an antiplatelet clotting effect (decreasing the risk of stroke) and tend to lower serum triglycerides and cholesterol. The fish of choice are those from cold water and the fatty fish such as salmon, herring, albacore tuna, mackerel, and sardines. You'll find quite a few tasty recipes for salmon and albacore tuna in this book!

Cut Cholesterol

Some people seem to be more sensitive to the cholesterol-raising effects of foods high in cholesterol than others. The food sources highest in dietary cholesterol are egg yolks, organ meats, especially liver, and whole-fat dairy products. I avoid organ meats altogether (which is usually not a problem for most people), I use egg substitutes whenever possible, and I buy only lower-fat milk, yogurt, and cheeses.

Glory in the Mysterious Influence of Fiber

There appears to be a way to have the best of both worlds. You can have the weight loss benefits (along with the blood pressure and blood cholesterol lowering benefits) of a high carbohydrate diet *and* the blood glucose, blood insulin, and serum triglyceride lowering benefits of a lower-carbohydrate diet. The answer is water-soluble fiber. Several studies have shown that the adverse metabolic effects of high-carbohydrate diets are neutralized when the high-carbohydrate diet is also high in fiber, particularly soluble fiber. These studies found that a high-carbohydrate and high-fiber diet improves blood glucose control, reduces plasma cholesterol, and at the same time, does *not* increase plasma insulin and serum triglycerides (as the high-carbohydrate diet might without the fiber).

Several studies have pointed the finger at the fiber in legumes (beans and peas), suggesting that this soluble fiber in particular lessens the negative metabolic side effects of high-carbohydrate diets. This is yet another reason to reach for beans.

There are many other reasons to emphasize soluble fibers in anyone's diet—with or without diabetes. For years water-soluble fibers have been linked to lowering serum cholesterol in the public at large; this is what gave oat bran its claim to fame. A recent six-year study of nearly 44,000 female health professionals reported that those who consumed the most fiber (25 grams or more per day) suffered 35 percent fewer heart attacks than those whose fiber was lowest. This and other studies have suggested that fiber helps protect against heart disease on its own, independent from the amount of fat or cholesterol in the diet. Imagine the protection if you put the two together—eat less fat and cholesterol in a diet that is rich in fiber.

How much fiber? Twenty-five grams or more per day seems to be the magic number. Dr. Eric Rimm, professor of epidemiology and nutrition at the Harvard School of Public Health, and others believe that this is the most protective level.

Get Your Vitamin E

Taking vitamin E supplements is associated with a reduced coronary risk. While I don't like an overreliance on diet supplements, I have to recognize that research keeps suggesting the importance of the unique antioxidant, vitamin E. Vitamin E appears to be the most potent antioxidant for LDL (bad cholesterol) oxidation. Regarding cancer prevention, vitamin E works like the other antioxidants, destroying oxygen-containing compounds, which can cause cancer if not kept in check. Vitamin E may even improve immune function, although more research needs to be done to confirm that benefit.

I usually steer away from nutrition recommendations that involve a vitamin pill and have a price tag attached to them. The overall nutrition picture usually fits neatly together: eat more fruits and vegetables and less animal fat, which can be done without turning to high-priced products. Mother Nature serves as our finest example of balance, moderation, and which nutrients tend to be particularly powerful. Except, it seems, when it comes to vitamin E—the antioxidant found primarily in plant oils.

It is impossible to consume vitamin E in the higher, seemingly beneficial amounts (100 to 400 I.U.) without the help of a supplement, especially if you are eating a low-fat, moderate-calorie diet.

More questions need to be answered. But until they are, it seems prudent to continue to emphasize food sources of vitamin E (vegetable oils except sesame, peanut, and olive oil, also kale, sweet potatoes, soybeans and tofu, nuts and almonds, and sunflower seeds). Taking a vitamin E supplement can also be considered—again, 100 I.U. is recommended as an effective and safe choice for most people.

Latch on to Folate (Folic Acid)—The Rising Star

The B vitamin folate is best known as a way to reduce the risk of neural tube defects in developing fetuses. But scores of recent studies have been showing us that's not all folate can do. A huge fifteen-year study of more than 5,000 men and women found that the lower the blood folate level, the higher the serum concentration of a chemical called homocysteine. That's not good because homocysteine seems to play a role in narrowing crucial arteries that circulate blood to the brain and heart—paving the way for future heart attacks or strokes.

Some researchers believe it is just as important to lower homocysteine levels as it is blood cholesterol. How much folate is enough to do the trick? Some folate researchers set the mark at 400 micrograms per day to maintain the blood levels of folate where they need to be to keep homocysteine levels low enough. Only 12 percent of Americans get this much folate in a day. The average American only gets half this amount (200 micrograms).

When you review the top folate food sources, it isn't hard to see why the average American diet comes up short. We don't tend to consume a lot of lentils and beans, orange juice, and green vegetables such as spinach, asparagus, and broccoli. But we should be eating more of these foods for other health reasons, which is one more reason to work them into our daily eating plan.

I make a point of drinking a glass of orange juice every morning, and I eat broccoli or a spinach salad almost every day. Also, I am constantly trying to eat more beans. This is one of my greatest food challenges, since many of the dishes I was raised on do not contain beans. But I love Mexican food, so I work them in here. And I love salads, so I add some there. It gets a little easier to eat beans every day.

Know the Exception to the Low-Fat, High-Carbohydrate Rule

There are conflicting reports of the metabolic impact of high-carbohydrate, low-fat diets on diabetics. A few researchers contend that the only data indicating low-fat, high-carbohydrate diets lead to beneficial effects on carbohydrate and lipoprotein metabolism are suspect, either because the diets differed in the type of dietary fat and amount of cholesterol consumed or because they were enormously enriched in dietary fiber, particularly water-soluble fiber.

The majority of researchers seem to think that a higher-fat diet is not in the long-term best interest of most people with Type II diabetes when there is a need for a decrease in body weight. Most researchers also agree that there will be exceptions to this rule. There will be circumstances when a particular person with Type II diabetes might manage his blood glucose and blood lipids better on a low-carbohydrate diet. People with hypertriglyceridemia, however, should probably not consider eating a diet that is too low in carbohydrate because it usually results in a much higher fat intake, which can lead to higher triglyceride levels throughout the day.

The person with Type II diabetes basically has two choices to reach good metabolic control: (1) a diet high in carbohydrate that is also high in dietary fiber (especially soluble fiber), or (2) a diet with a higher fat total (although saturated fat is still low) and a lower carbohydrate total. In this second option, the increase in fat should come from the monounsaturated fats, and fiber should still be adequate.

Be Aware of the Genetics, Diet, and Coronary Heart Disease Connections

As a person with diabetes, you need to be aware of any additional personal factors that would predispose you to heart disease. Genetics are one factor. We all know that if we have heart disease in our family, it increases our risk of contracting heart disease. But by how much? I've always found this issue personally interesting since my family history and Dutch heritage are riddled with heart attacks and strokes. My maternal grandfather and his four brothers all died of heart attacks or strokes around their fiftieth birthday. If that isn't having heart disease in your family, I don't know what is!

Half of the American population's fluctuation in both good (HDL) and bad (LDL) cholesterol levels is thought to be caused by genetics—primarily affecting our lipoproteins and their receptors. People who inherit the "normal" lipoprotein processes tend to have normal serum lipoprotein levels until middle age. After this point, their lipoproteins may rise because of diabetes, obesity, lack of exercise, or a diet high in fat, especially saturated fat. But the person who inherits the "flawed" lipoprotein mechanisms may start to show abnormal blood lipids and signs of atherosclerosis at an earlier age.

Genetics may also determine the particle size of our LDL cholesterol, and LDL particle size may encourage atherosclerosis. In this case bigger is better. There is some evidence that small, dense LDL particles are the most likely to oxidize and damage the arteries. The genetic tendency to produce smaller LDL particles is thought to affect one out of every four Americans, placing them at higher risk of coronary heart disease.

Research also indicates that increasing or decreasing cholesterol or saturated fat in our diet will result in a wide range of blood lipid responses across the population. Some people show big changes in their serum cholesterol after dietary cholesterol and saturated fat have been increased or decreased, while others show almost no change at all. But for the people with a genetic tendency toward abnormal blood lipid levels, a low-fat diet with a higher ratio of unsaturated fats to saturated fats seems to invoke the most dramatic improvements.

Now that you know more than you ever thought you wanted to know about glucose, lipids, and the related health terrors for people with diabetes—how do you use this information to manage your condition and stay healthy? Let's look at our four strategies and how they fit together with the right attitude.

STRATEGY #1: MODERATE WEIGHT LOSS

What does obesity have to do with Type II diabetes? A whole lot—for most. Obesity is clearly one factor that causes the insulin resistance typical in Type II diabetes. So if obesity can help cause diabetes, can losing weight help control diabetes? You bet.

Losing 10 to 20 pounds, considered "moderate" weight loss, has been shown to improve many things that diabetics care about: namely, it reduces elevated blood glucose, abnormal lipid levels (dyslipidemia), and high blood pressure (hypertension)—no matter what the starting weight. Plasma triglycerides are also likely to decline when people lose weight and rise when they gain weight—regardless of the food they are eating. By losing some weight, you can actually make your cells more sensitive to insulin (whether the insulin comes from your pancreas or an injection). Losing 10 to 20 pounds can be pretty powerful stuff.

Losing a little "around the middle" can be especially beneficial because it is abdominal obesity in particular that is associated with the metabolic diseases (i.e., Type II diabetes, impaired glucose tolerance, high blood pressure, and lipid abnormalities). The ratio of your waist and hip circumference is a strong risk factor for Type II diabetes in both men and women. In fact, a recent study statistically showed that insulin resistance is more closely associated with abdominal obesity (also known as girth) than with age.

You can discover your abdominal obesity, if you dare, with only a simple measuring tape. Measure your waist and your hips in inches. Divide your waist measurement by your hip measurement. A fraction >.95 for men, >.8 for women indicates risk for metabolic diseases. I think this is the most valuable way to gauge your progress as you begin adopting a new eating plan and exercise schedule. As long as your fraction is moving in the right direction (down), you are on the road to improving your health risk.

For example, if your waist is 45 inches and your hips are 45 inches, the fraction is 1.0. But if your waist pares down to 40 inches and your hips to 44 inches, your new fraction is .9 and your abdominal obesity has decreased.

Are You Wearing the Fat Gene?

Are you wearing the fat gene? I know I am. It isn't difficult to figure this one out. Look up your family tree for a few generations. Were your mom, dad, or grandparents a little "fluffy" or were they "string beans"? Did the women resemble "pears" or "apples" when they put on a little extra weight? If string beans *and* apples are both growing on your family tree, then it's the luck of the draw. My grandparents on both sides were each split green beans and apples. But both my parents, as luck would have it, received the apple gene. Guess what happened to me and my two sisters? Let's put it this way—none of us are string beans. You've heard about (or maybe witnessed) how some people can eat and eat and eat and never get fat? Well, these people probably don't have the fat gene.

I remember learning years ago about how when groups of mice were given a marginally adequate amount of food, there was little difference in their size. But when an excess of food was given, particularly fat calories, certain strains of mice became much fatter than others. So it makes sense then that a genetic predisposition to chubbiness may determine how our body handles calorie and fat excess more than anything else. It seems that in a society like ours, where inactivity and a high-fat diet are the norm, you are more likely to see big differences in body shapes and sizes.

The fat gene research has gotten a lot more sophisticated. Molecular geneticists have identified the gene that, when mutated, causes a severe hereditary obesity in mice. They also discovered that humans have a very similar gene to the mouse obesity gene. This may be the gene whose role is to regulate the size of the body's fat stores. It has also been suggested that this gene may act on the body by releasing a hormone of some kind.

Earlier research proved the hypothalamus (a part of the brain) to be important for controlling food intake and energy expenditure, two ways the body regulates fat deposition. We have only scratched the fat gene surface; there is a lot more to learn. Some scientists predict that obesity is influenced by a variety of genes working in tandem. Perhaps the fat genes act some way on the hypothalamus.

While it is true your genetic background helps determine your future chances of becoming overweight or obese, genetics tell only part of the story. You see, experts estimate body weight is 40 to 70 percent heritable—which means you can look at this fat gene two ways. The glass can be half empty or half full. I see the 40 to 70 percent as definitely leaving the door open for lifestyle choices. You may never be a string bean, but you can be a fit and shapely apple.

Where Do You Wear Your Extra Fat?

Do you wear your fat around the middle? Does your shape resemble an apple or a pear? These are very important questions because it is extra abdominal fat (the apples) that appears to encourage insulin resistance more so than fat on other parts of the body (such as the thigh and buttocks area—the pear). Abdominal obesity, independent of total fat mass, also increases your risk of cardiovascular disease, stroke, and hypertension. And guess what, you may also have your mom or dad to thank for this. Studies in genetic epidemiology have shown that the total amount of body fat and the way your body distributes that fat have powerful genetic influences.

I know firsthand what it is like to live in an apple-shaped physique that, despite my daily efforts, appears to be preprogrammed for extra padding—complete with a low metabolic rate. I have to work hard at staying only slightly overweight. I exercise every day, eat lower-fat foods, and I never overeat. My prize?—Staying a size 12 to 14. (For male readers: that's a well-rounded medium, approaching large.) But you know what my real prize is? I feel great, I have a lot of energy, and my body is well conditioned and fit. I don't care what size you are, eating healthy foods and getting fit with regular exercise makes you feel great. And that's the best reason of all to improve your lifestyle.

Right now, though, how you collected the extra weight over the years or even how many pounds overweight you are are less important. I don't want you to focus on how much weight you are losing. Instead, I want you to shift your focus from "weight" to "good health"—from feeling "bad" or "wanting to be thin" to feeling "healthy"—from "deprivation" to "moderation." Concentrate on the same things I would tell a person of normal weight to concentrate on:

- Eat a nutritious, low-fat diet (see chapters 5 and 6 for more on this).
- Learn to eat when you are hungry and stop when you are comfortable; avoid starving yourself and overeating (see chapter 6 for more on appetite and overeating).
- Get regular exercise (see Strategy #3 for more on exercise).

These are keys to having a healthier lifestyle for everyone, not just those with diabetes, and not just people who are overweight. These three keys help lower your risk for such serious illnesses as cancer, heart disease, and high blood pressure. If you shed some pounds by improving your lifestyle, then that's a bonus!

Weight Loss with Insulin

It seems painfully ironic that insulin is often given to overweight people with Type II diabetes when insulin could, by anyone's standard, be considered "fattening." It increases your appetite, and it encourages your body to deposit fat stores.

So, you are told to take your insulin, which for many people is the only medication that may help them control their blood sugar at that point in their diabetes, but at the same time, you are also told to eat less food (if weight loss is one of your treatment goals) *and* lose weight.

What can we learn from this? First, you might avoid insulin as long as you can. Second, if you are on insulin, understand that it may be even more difficult to lose weight. So, don't concentrate on the pounds gained or lost, which could be very discouraging. And what do many people do when they feel discouraged? They tend to eat for comfort and give up on many of the healthful habits they have been following thus far. Feeling discouraged will only make things worse.

In fact, put your scale away. Instead, concentrate on what you *do* have some control over—following your eating and exercise plan as best you can. The numbers to watch are your blood sugar numbers. Are they going down? This is a great way for you to measure your success.

If you are overweight, part of your therapy will probably include moderate weight loss via moderate calorie restriction (Strategy #2), regular exercise (Strategy #3), and a meal plan that follows the diet recommendations. But there are a couple things people with Type II diabetes on insulin need to do that other Type IIs don't—synchronizing meal size and times to the time actions of insulin is one. Monitoring blood glucose levels frequently is another. You can work with your diabetes health care team to make appropriate insulin adjustments based on blood glucose patterns that may arise.

Burning More Calories

When we are advised to shed some pounds we are always told to eat less or to take in fewer calories (there is more on cutting calories in Strategy #2 following). But one of the best strategies for losing weight is the other side of the food equation—burning *more* calories. The most direct way to encourage your body to use more calories is to exercise (Strategy #3). Not only do you burn calories to fuel your body while you are exercising, but your body also tends to burn more calories than it normally would *after* the exercise. Strength training, in particular, helps you build muscle. And the more muscle you have, the more calories you burn—even when you are resting. Pretty great, isn't it! Studies show that people derive these benefits with just two strength-training sessions a week.

Another way to burn more calories is to eat smaller, more frequent meals (this is Strategy #4). Each time you eat, you start the digestive/absorptive process going. It takes some calories just to start it up and more calories to keep it going. So the more times you get it started and going, the more calories you are likely to burn digesting your food.

Eating a high-carbohydrate diet versus a high-fat diet is also likely to burn more calories. Your body uses more energy (burns more calories) metabolizing carbohydrate than it does breaking down fat and storing it as body fat. It appears the human body has several hormonal systems in place to help handle bigger influxes of carbohydrate and protein calories; in contrast, the body does not seem to have any such system for fat.

A Tale of Two Dieters

Tanya cut her calories back, like most people who diet. She ate about 500 fewer calories each day than normal. And she lost more than 8 pounds in six months. But Tanya was irritable through much of these six months. She was tired of counting calories and tired of feeling hungry.

Linda cut her fat intake to about 20 grams a day. She didn't count calories, so she didn't know she was eating about 400 fewer calories a day than normal. She ate small servings of meat and whatever complex carbohydrates she wanted. She lost almost 10 pounds in six months. Linda was happier eating this way than Tanya was on her calorie-counting plan. Linda felt that she was eating food she liked and didn't have many cravings. She also thought she had more energy and believed she would keep eating this way in the future.

Denver is one city, and there are many roads that lead to Denver. Well, there are many ways to lose weight. If you are smart, you will choose the road (or eating plan) that is more scenic, more interesting, and the most enjoyable. The University of Minnesota placed 122 moderately overweight women on one of the two diet methods described above with Tanya and Linda. They discovered that the less fat the women ate, and the heavier they were at the start of the study, the more weight they lost. The calories seemed to be less important.

STRATEGY #2:   CUTTING CALORIES

"Restricting calories"—boy, I hate the sound of that. So I changed it to "cutting calories," which somehow doesn't sound as bad. A moderate calorie restriction, described as 500 to 1,000 calories less than the usual daily intake, along with a nutritionally adequate meal plan, is usually encouraged for overweight Type IIs. Another way to look at this task is to calculate what your calorie needs are, based on a realistic weight goal.

You can measure your usual calorie intake by analyzing your current diet; chapter 5 will show you how. Subtract about 500 calories from that figure if a moderate cut in calories is in order.

ARE YOU OVEREATING?

Do you eat when you are *not* really hungry? If you do, why do you think you do this? Out of stress? Boredom? Because you feel deprived? Because you want to be sociable? If you tend to eat when you are under stress or bored, for instance, try to relax another way. Take a walk, turn on your favorite music, or seek one of the many forms of diversion available today. Once you've determined whether or not you are truly hungry, the next question is Do you often overeat?

Habitual overeating (that is, eating many more calories than your body actually needs) is thought to increase the risk of macrovascular disease. Since many Type II people are also trying to trim off a few extra pounds, eating just until you are comfortably full (or not hungry anymore) is great.

How can you avoid the urge to overeat? One of the best ways I know of is to avoid getting overly hungry. That is, don't deprive yourself completely either in a social setting or during your daily routine. For example, many experts believe a morning meal helps prevent late-day overeating. If you skip breakfast, you may be more likely to overeat at lunch and maybe even dinner. And if you skip lunch as well, you are almost guaranteed to eat through the late afternoon and evening to compensate.

Another way to avoid overeating is to sit down, relax, eat slowly, and stick with small portions. Give your stomach some time to tell your brain that it is comfortably full.

I think people overeat sometimes because what they have been eating isn't satisfying or enjoyable. Try to choose foods that you like and look forward to and that fit into your eating plan. If you love fettuccine Alfredo, find a tasty low-fat way to make it, then enjoy it. If you feel like something chocolate, get yourself a little piece of chocolate and be done with it. Otherwise, you might get increasingly interested in eating chocolate until you finally let yourself have some and eat five times as much as you would have otherwise.

That Amazing Shrinking Stomach

Is it just me or does everyone wake up ravenous after eating more than usual the night before? You'd think you would be *less* hungry the morning after. But if your stomach has been stretched, because you overate, it can actually feel more empty than usual the next day after all the food has been digested. This is just one example of the amazing shrinking—and expanding—stomach.

Researchers recently measured the holding capacity of obese people's stomachs before and after participating in a weight-loss regimen. Before the diet, the participants could hold an average of 4 cups of water in their stomachs. Four weeks later, and after losing 12 to 28 pounds, their stomachs could hold an average of less than 3 cups of water.

The researchers suggest that eating overly large individual meals increases stomach capacity more than eating too many calories over the course of a day. But here's the clincher: the larger the holding capacity of the stomach, the easier it is to eat a large meal and the greater your desire to eat a large meal. You can thank "stretching sensors" in your stomach for this.

When stretched sufficiently, stretching sensors in the stomach send signals to the brain to induce satiety or fullness. The sensors may not start sending signals until the stomach has distended to a certain proportion of its capacity. Therefore, the smaller the stomach's holding capacity, the sooner it will inform the brain (and the smaller the amount of food necessary) that it is comfortably full.

STRATEGY #3:   EXERCISE

I have always said I would rather dance for three hours than run for thirty minutes. That's because I hate running and I love dancing. Thirty minutes of doing something you don't like can seem like three hours, while three hours of something you love and think is fun can seem like thirty minutes—so choose something you like or love. I love Jazzercise. And I've been doing it three times a week, faithfully, for seven years. I like my treadmill a lot less. How often do I work out using it? Twice a month. You need to exercise more than twice a month.

The Dynamic Duo—Eating Healthy and Exercise

For almost every major chronic disease, exercise goes hand-in-hand with a healthy diet. Exercise will help you lose weight, which will help improve your blood sugar and blood lipids. But exercise also helps improve your blood sugar more directly. Exercise improves the muscle cells' ability to take in and use glucose, so it makes insulin-resistant cells less resistant. Exercise also helps reduce your risk of heart disease and helps lower your blood pressure and cholesterol levels, which all people with Type II diabetes need to watch carefully, considering their increased risk of heart disease.

Start Exercising Yesterday

There are seven great reasons to exercise; some offer short-term rewards, and some long-term rewards. Right away, exercising will start helping you feel better about yourself and will help you cope with stress. And right away you will seem to have more energy throughout the day. Also, right from the start, exercise will help your body use insulin better. If you keep at it, you can look forward to several other health benefits. Exercise keeps you flexible and strong, exercise helps you maintain or arrive at a healthier weight, and exercise helps lower your blood glucose, blood cholesterol, and blood pressure.

How and When to Exercise

What: Exercise is anything that gets your heart beating and uses the large muscles in your legs and arms. Walking is probably the easiest form of exercise for most people. But you may enjoy an aerobics class, swimming, water aerobics, chair aerobics, bike riding, rowing, or dancing. If you know you probably won't stick with exercise unless you have an exercise companion, choose a form of exercise that involves a class, or ask a friend to exercise with you.

How long: Start with five minutes and work up to twenty to thirty minutes if you can.

How often: Exercise every day, if possible, but at least three times a week.

How hard: Work with your health care team on your target heart rate. As a rule, you should feel a little winded, but you should be able to talk while you are exercising.

When: The best time to exercise is 1 to $1^1/2$ hours after a meal. Work with your health care team to find the best fit for exercise in your schedule.

Planning for Exercise

Exercise acts as an insulin enhancer; it tends to lower blood sugar. In fact, blood sugar can continue to decrease for up to twelve to twenty-four hours after the exercise session is over. However, every individual responds differently. Any adjustments in food intake or insulin must be based on blood sugar levels and how your exercise has affected you before. *In general,* figure you'll need 10 to 15 grams of carbohydrate after every hour of exercise. The key is to monitor your blood sugar before and after in order to track how a particular exercise (and of what duration) affects you and whether a snack after exercise is necessary.

People with Type II diabetes who are *not* obese probably need to pay the most attention to adjusting their meal plan to compensate for their exercise sessions. Usually Type IIs being treated with diet alone or oral hypoglycemics do not need supplementary food when exercising.

Plan ahead to work in your scheduled exercise efficiently. Keep your workout shoes and clothes in your car or briefcase if you exercise outside the home. Pack a snack or high-sugar food such as juice in case you have a low blood sugar reaction.

Finally, as always, check with your doctor before you begin a new exercise program. Talk to her about consulting an exercise physiologist who understands the special problems of having diabetes. If you must, health team captain, find an expert on you own.

STRATEGY #4:   EATING SMALLER, MORE FREQUENT MEALS

Eating more often, but smaller amounts at a time, may be just what the doctored ordered, particularly for people with Type II diabetes. Smaller meals spaced throughout the day have resulted in smaller blood glucose responses and required less insulin, improving blood glucose control in recent studies on Type II people. Another study demonstrated that the closer together the meals were, the better the glucose tolerance.

This makes sense to me because the bigger the meal, the larger the number of calories eaten from carbohydrate, fat, and protein, and the higher the blood levels of those nutrients after the meal.

Smaller, lower-fat meals will not stay as long in the stomach before moving on to the intestines, leaving you more energetic after eating. A larger meal might leave you sleepy, lowering the calories you might otherwise be burning if you felt active and were moving around. This eating pattern also helps keep us from getting overly hungry, which can lead to overeating or poor food choices.

One research team even demonstrated a reduction of heart disease in the people who ate more frequently. Eating eight meals a day or more was effective in lowering serum cholesterol, compared to the standard three meals a day. Lowering your serum cholesterol and improving your blood glucose control aren't the only reasons to eat smaller, more frequent meals. Another study observed that obesity was less common in people who ate more frequent meals.

If you are going to eat the standard three meals a day, the prevailing wisdom would be to space them out at four- to five-hour intervals. In fact, experts have not yet determined the ideal eating pattern for people with diabetes. The best choice right now: space your meals according to your individual schedule, blood glucose goals, ability to handle food intake, and so on.

ATTITUDE ADJUSTMENT: GETTING YOUR MIND RIGHT

You've no doubt noticed that the four strategies for achieving the twin goals of controlling blood glucose and blood lipids levels are tightly interwoven. You lose weight by cutting calories and burning calories more efficiently through exercise and the proper spacing of meals.

You've probably also observed that the strategies not only involve what you do but how you think. I stressed while talking about weight loss, for instance, the need to refocus your efforts on being healthy and feeling good rather than dropping pounds. The same attitude adjustment applies when figuring out how to cut calories, when to eat, and the how, where, when, and what to do about exercise.

Think health. Think control. Yes, think freedom. Taking charge of your diet, your schedule, your activities is liberating. You are doing something for yourself. As a matter of fact, you are doing several things for yourself. You are achieving the keys to success I mentioned in chapter 1—monitoring blood levels, exercising, and following a diet plan.

A positive outlook also comes from enjoying the process. I have already given you a lot of good news about the food you can eat, and much more is on the way in the remaining chapters. I'll have advice on meal planning that will make Strategies #1, #2, and #4 a lot easier to swallow. As for Strategy #3, exercise, I can only repeat: Find some activities you enjoy and, perhaps, people you enjoy doing them with. Please remember, health team captain, you have experts and friends you can go to for advice and support.

PART TWO

THE GOOD NEWS
EATING PLAN

5

THE C-F-F GRAM-COUNTING PLAN

Counting and categorizing every morsel that goes in your mouth is, at the very least, tiresome. For people with diabetes, it may feel as if they're being punished for having a disease. Speaking personally and professionally as a dietitian, I hate the idea of counting nutrients every time I sit down to eat. However, I realize that, for people with diabetes, the physical benefits probably outweigh the psychological anguish. My aim is to help assemble an eating plan that you can live happily with, one that maximizes the health benefits from counting and minimizes the feelings of punishment and monotony.

There are many meal-planning systems and guides for people with diabetes to choose from. The "food group" plan promotes balance, while the "carbo blocks" and "carbo counting" plans keep track of carbohydrates only. The age-old "exchange system" does both by telling you how much to eat of each food group during each meal or snack. The exchange system is probably the most structured of all the eating plans. I can remember learning the exchange system fifteen years ago in my college nutrition classes. Even then I found it complicated and constricting.

Which eating plan is best for you? The decision is yours. Which do you feel most comfortable with? Which method matches your personal lifestyle and food choices the best? For the purposes of this book, which is written for food-loving people with Type II diabetes, I had to use at least one of these eating plans as a guide for the recipes and meal examples, and as a way for you to evaluate other meals you prepare and those you eat out. What follows is how I arrived at a general plan that is likely to work for you.

Even though I've heard some diabetes specialists refer to carbo counting as a method more for Type I people, it's the one I prefer and the method most preferred by the Type IIs I spoke with. Counting *carbohydrate grams* may be considered severe or overkill for Type IIs not on insulin, but many Type IIs

69

will eventually end up on insulin to control their blood sugar. Wouldn't it be better to start off with *one* manageable eating plan that will take you through all possible stages of diabetes? Further, since many Type IIs are probably going to count *fat grams*, to aid in the weight loss effort and to help reduce risk of heart disease, why not count carbohydrates the same way—grams?

Some of the food plans focus on carbohydrates, emphasizing blood sugar control; some focus on counting fat in efforts to lower lipid levels and aid in weight loss; still others consider calories to encourage modest weight loss. Wouldn't it be best to combine all of these into one system? After all, most people with Type II diabetes are concerned about blood sugar control, reducing their risk of heart disease, *and* losing a little weight if possible.

If many people with diabetes are counting fat grams as part of a low-fat diet, they are probably opting for the high-carbohydrate eating plan. And in order to consume this diet without the negative blood sugar and blood lipid effects (which accompany the high-carbohydrate diet for many of those with diabetes), they will also need to eat a high-*fiber* diet (primarily soluble fiber). Which means they might also benefit from counting *grams of fiber*.

So, there you have it. The C-F-F Gram-Counting Plan. You count grams of *C*arbohydrates, *F*at, and *F*iber. I hope this is a system that can serve you over many years—whether you start taking insulin, whether you start showing signs of heart disease, or whether you decide to opt for the higher-fat, lower-carbohydrate plan. Either way you are counting carbohydrates either to keep them low, balance them with your insulin, or spread them evenly throughout the day. Either way you are counting fat to make sure you have enough, but not too much. Either way you are counting fiber to make sure you have enough. Even if you opt for the lower-carbohydrate, higher-fat eating plan, fiber will still benefit your health and should still be consumed in adequate amounts.

Before we get into the details of C-F-F counting, I want to discuss how to determine the quantity to eat at a sitting.

PORTION SIZE SUCCESS

If your food portions are too large, your blood glucose will be higher than your goal, and you may even gain weight. If you take diabetes medicine or insulin, your blood glucose may go too low if your portions are too small or too high if your portions are too large. You see, you are keeping track of your food portions not only to make sure you don't have too much, but also to make sure you are getting enough.

If you are like many Type IIs, making sure your portions are just right will probably be your greatest dietary challenge. But your greatest challenge can also be your fastest way to blood glucose success. Keeping portions moderate is thought to be the single most important aspect in meal planning for blood glucose control. How do you make sure your portion sizes are moderate? In a word—measuring. Measuring and counting your food before a meal is the best way to guarantee portion size sucess.

Now, I know measuring food can be everything from tedious to embarrassing. Even if your meal plan is providing enough food to satisfy your hunger, measuring food, in and of itself, can make you feel deprived or punished. Try to focus on the positive part of measuring. This is a tool to improve your blood sugar. Use it; make it work for you. And it's not forever. Eventually, after several weeks of measuring food, you will become an expert portion estimator. You will be able to eyeball proper portions of food with acceptable accuracy.

Generally speaking, you use liquid measuring cups to measure liquids and dry measuring cups and measuring spoons to measure solids. You can use a food scale to weigh foods in ounces or grams. Here's a guide to help you match the best measuring method to the food:

Use a *scale* to measure the *weight* of
baked goods (cornbread, muffins, date-nut bread, rolls, etc.)
baked potatoes
bread, roll, bagel
fruits that vary in size (bananas, apples)
meats

Use measuring cups and spoons to measure the *volume* of
beverages
casseroles
cereals
condiments
fruits that come in pieces (grapes, berries)
mixed dishes
noodles
rice
soups
vegetables and mashed potatoes

Sometimes you are just going to have to eyeball it and estimate the portion size, especially when you are eating out. A 3-ounce serving of cooked

Let Your Hand Be Your Guide

When measuring cups or spoons are nowhere in sight, you can estimate serving sizes using your hand. These comparisons are based on an average-size woman's hand.

Your thumb	=	1 ounce of cheese
The tip of your thumb	=	1 teaspoon
(three thumb tips	=	1 tablespoon)
Your fist	=	1 cup
The palm of your hand	=	3 ounces of meat

meat is about the size of a deck of playing cards or the palm of your hand, for example. See chart, "Let Your Hand Be Your Guide," above.

As intimidating as this sounds, take heart. The more practice you have, the better you will become at estimating portion sizes, and you won't have to measure everything all of the time.

Consider also that most of us buy the same food products in the grocery store every week. Most of us eat the same ten recipes repeatedly. Most people order the same items at their favorite restaurants. Once you have measured amounts and counted up the carbohydrates, fat, and fiber to find the right fit, you don't have to do it again. You will already know how much is best when you are having that particular meal. You will already know that you can order a certain dish when you are at a particular restaurant or fast food chain. Because you have added everything up before. Because you tested your blood sugar after having that same meal several times before.

Your Eyes May Be Bigger Than Your Measuring Cup

Test your portion size perception. Measure out certain basic portions of food using your trained eye. Guesstimate how much 1 cup of cold cereal is, for example, while pouring it into a bowl. Or cut what you think is 2 ounces of cheese. Now put those foods to the test. Use measuring cups, spoons, or the scale to measure how much it really is. Is it more or less than the serving you thought it was? How close did you come?

Label Mathematics

The Nutrition Facts panel on the new food label lists a serving size and the number of servings in the package. It also lists the number of calories, carbohydrates, fat, and fiber in one serving of the food. All right, that's pretty straightforward, but here's the tricky part: the serving size on the food label may not be exactly the amount of food you like to eat in one serving. And it also may not be what you think one serving of that food is. You may think a serving of ice cream is 1 cup. But the ice cream companies think a serving is half that much. You may think two cookies is a serving. They may think a serving is only one cookie. You might assume that one Snickers bar is one serving; they think it is two servings. Don't assume. Always check the label. You might be surprised.

The number of servings per package can also get a little complicated. A can of soup, for example, may contain 2.5 servings, according to the label. So if you eat the whole can, you'll need to multiply the calories and grams of carbohydrates, fat, and fiber by 2.5. Life would be simpler if the numbers were nice and neat all of the time, but they're not.

Be prepared to read some labels and perform some simple math functions in the C-F-F Gram Counting Plan. If you like to use 3 tablespoons of a certain salad dressing on your salad, but the Nutrition Facts label on the bottle lists 1 serving as 2 tablespoons, you'll need to multiply the calories and grams of carbohydrate and fat by 1.5 (3 tablespoons divided by 2 tablespoons is 1.5). If you like to eat three slices of Louis Rich Turkey Bacon with breakfast, you will need to multiply the calories and fat by 3, since the label lists this information per 1 slice. See the table below for the calculations.

Basic Label Math

For 3 slices of Louis Rich Turkey Bacon, triple the totals

	The label says		*Your total is*
Calories	30	× 3	90
Total fat	2.5 g	× 3	7.5 g
Saturated fat	0.5 g	× 3	1.5 g
Cholesterol	10 mg	× 3	30 mg
Carbohydrate	0 g		0
Fiber	0 g		0

COUNTING CARBOHYDRATES

Carbohydrates may not be the enemy, but they are, most definitely, the first beast you must tame. It is the carbohydrate in food that has the most influence on blood glucose levels. Protein and fat in food do not raise blood glucose nearly as high as carbohydrates. That's why, in terms of blood glucose levels, counting carbohydrates and eating nearly the same amounts of carbohydrate each day are most important.

Carbohydrate Food Sources

Most people know that fruit, breads, and sugars are big carbohydrate contributors. Other carbohydrate sources are crackers, cereals, pasta, rice, and other grain products; starchy vegetables; milk and yogurt; fruit juice; and any sweetener such as sugar, honey, syrups, and molasses.

Some carbohydrate-rich foods are also rich in protein—for example, peas and beans, milk and yogurt. But it is fat, not protein, that goes along with the carbohydrate in many of our *favorite* foods, such as cakes, pies, cookies, chocolate, ice cream, and chips.

Getting your "5 a Day" (5 servings of fruits and vegetables) is a great goal, even if you don't have diabetes. Always try to include at least 3 vegetable servings and 2 fruit servings in your carbohydrate total each day. These carbohydrate sources contribute valuable vitamins, minerals, and phytochemicals, as well as fiber.

In terms of blood sugar, are all carbohydrate-rich foods created equal? Probably not. Then are some carbohydrate-rich foods better choices than others in terms of blood sugar? Possibly. It appears that some foods, when the same amount of carbohydrate is eaten, can raise or lower your blood sugar levels after you eat. This variation is measured by the glycemic index, which I discussed at length in the previous chapter.

As I mentioned in chapter 4, there are many studies of the glycemic index of carbohydrate-rich foods; most have validated the concept that some carbohydrate-rich foods affect blood sugar differently from others. The results are predictable even when mixed meals are eaten. The index is therefore reliable and useful in dietary management of both diabetes and hyperlipidemia (high blood lipid levels). To that end, authors of a recent journal article brought together all of the quality published data on the glycemic index of individual foods to make one comprehensive glycemic index table. You will find this listing of foods with their glycemic indexes, from low to high, in chapter 6.

Timing Is Important

When and how often you consume your carbohydrate grams is also important. For example, many people with diabetes are more sensitive to carbohydrate foods first thing in the morning. Your dietitian or diabetes educator might work with you to set a smaller number of carbohydrate grams as your target for breakfast compared to your other meals.

And obviously, eating your daily allotment of grams of carbohydrate in one sitting isn't the idea either. Spacing your carbohydrate foods out over the day is a crucial part of carbo-counting success. Even if you don't take insulin or diabetes pills, spacing carbohydrates makes it easier for your body's insulin to work on the glucose it is getting from food.

Your dietitian or diabetes educator will work with you to set carbohydrate gram goals for each meal or snack time. Once the goals are set, your experience will tell you whether they need to be adjusted up or down. This is called fine-tuning. As the days go by and you continue to eat according to your carbohydrate gram goals, test your blood sugar, take any prescribed medication, and stick to your exercise plan. You and your health care team will be able to see whether it's working. Do you feel good? Is your blood sugar improved? Are there trouble spots—times of day when your blood sugar is consistently high or low?

Carbohydrate Counting 101

The carbohydrate content of a food is always measured in grams (g), a unit of weight in the metric system. The grams of carbohydrate should not be confused with the weight of the overall food. The grams of carbohydrate are the measure of the food's carbohydrate content; the gram measure of the overall food is how much the food physically weighs. For example, a serving of a particular food may weigh 200 grams and have 25 grams of carbohydrate.

You may want to know how a gram compares to an ounce: A gram is $1/28$ of an ounce, or 1 ounce is equal to 28 grams. (One gram is the weight of a standard paper clip.)

How Close Do You Need to Come to Your Carbohydrate Target?

It is up to you and your dietitian or certified diabetes educator to determine how close you need to come to your carbohydrate target for each meal. In general, the American Diabetes Association urges people with diabetes to stay within 5 grams (plus or minus) of their carbohydrate goal at each meal or snack.

COUNTING FAT

Heart disease, cancer, and possible weight gain are three good reasons to count fat grams, because too much fat, especially saturated fat, will increase your risk for all three. While counting carbohydrates offers the person with diabetes eating-plan flexibility, focusing only on carbohydrates and ignoring protein and fat could increase the risk of weight gain.

A high-fat meal or high-fat and high-protein meal can also slow down the time your stomach takes to empty. This may delay your after-meal rise in blood sugar levels. You might notice that your bedtime blood glucose is higher than usual following a high-fat dinner. That's one of the reasons why I like the C-F-F Gram counting plan. It doesn't ignore fat—it includes it.

Even if you normally eat low-fat meals, you will no doubt encounter those unavoidable or irresistible high-fat meals such as barbecued ribs and French fries or fettuccine Alfredo from a restaurant or a high-fat and high-protein meal such as prime rib. If you take insulin, your dietitian or diabetes educator can show you how to make adjustments in the dose or timing of your insulin for those occasional high-fat meals.

What's Your Target Number of Fat Grams?

Most people with diabetes need some fat in every meal or snack to help slow down the digestive process a little and to help balance the carbohydrate. I also think a little fat in every meal helps us feel satisfied and in many cases makes the meal more enjoyable. How much fat? Now there's the billion-dollar question.

As I pointed out earlier, there is a difference of opinion among diabetes researchers about whether a low-fat, high-carbohydrate diet or a low-carbohydrate diet (high monounsaturated fat) is better for most people with Type II diabetes. The answer may be right inside your own body. You need to know which eating plan your own personal blood sugar and blood lipids respond to best.

So, to give you some ballpark figures of how many grams of fat your daily target might be, I calculated grams of fat per day per a given number of daily calories for three different eating plans. In the table on page 80 you can see what the fat gram target is at the 1,800 calorie level, for example, for 25 percent calories from fat (50 grams), 35 percent calories from fat (70 grams), and 40 percent calories from fat (80 grams).

The higher the percentage of calories from fat, and as the fat gram targets increase, the food sources of those fats become even more important. Saturated fat should remain low. The monounsaturated fats should provide the bulk of the fat grams. For more information on emphasizing monounsaturated fats and limiting saturated fat, see tips and tables in chapter 6 and recipes in chapter 8.

COUNTING FIBER

When you think of fiber, you might think of the words, "roughage," "bulk," or "bran." People usually know that fiber keeps food waste moving through the intestines swiftly, thereby preventing the dreaded "c" word—*constipation*. Fiber does this because it isn't digested by the human body; therefore, it cannot be absorbed into the bloodstream like other carbohydrates and travels through the entire intestinal tract intact. That's right, fiber is considered a carbohydrate—it is simply a carbohydrate that cannot be digested. So it is logical that fiber does not become blood glucose. But this is not to say that fiber does not *affect* blood glucose. In fact, your blood glucose may be *lower* after a high-fiber meal than after a low-fiber meal.

The benefits of eating a lot of fiber are still being studied. But so far, it appears that fiber reduces the amount of calories we tend to consume (in part by increasing the bulkiness of food and by increasing the immediate sense of fullness) and slows down stomach emptying. And last but not least, a high-fiber eating plan seems to improve glycemic (blood sugar) control. One study on people with Type II diabetes consuming a high-soluble-fiber diet actually showed a reduction of insulin requirements by 75 to 100 percent. Some participants were able to get off insulin completely. The effect of fiber seems to be pretty powerful. Studies have also shown that fiber taken at one meal has a beneficial effect on glucose tolerance in subsequent meals.

The high-fiber eating plan seems to be more effective at lowering postmeal glucose levels than at lowering morning fasting glucose levels. But don't we spend at least half of each day in a postmeal state rather than a fasting state?

The same study mentioned above of people with Type II diabetes also showed a reduction of serum cholesterol by 24 percent (the effects on serum triglycerides varied). *Soluble fiber* is thought to help reduce serum lipids probably by binding with cholesterol-containing bile acids (secreted by the large intestines to aid in digestion) and carrying them out of the body, along with other waste. In the process, the fiber also seems to reduce the absorption of some of the food fat also present in the intestines. A fall in HDL cholesterol might be observed once a high-carbohydrate, high-fiber diet is adopted, but researchers have observed this effect to be short-term, with original levels returning after six months.

Getting some fiber, especially soluble fiber, in every meal is a great goal for the Type IIs. How much fiber? Well, as I mentioned in chapter 4, the general public is urged by various dietary guidelines and health agencies to consume about 25 to 30 grams of fiber a day. Some diabetes researchers suggest 30 or 40 grams of fiber for the person with diabetes.

I'll admit, it isn't easy to reach even the 30 or more grams of fiber a day target. But it isn't impossible either. Work with your dietitian or diabetes educator to come up with some fiber goals for each meal. For example, you might aim for 12 grams of fiber in your breakfast and 9 grams each at lunch and dinner.

You might want to try boosting your soluble fiber during the time of day when your blood sugar is harder to control or during meals that tend to raise your blood sugar. For example, if your blood sugar tends to rise higher than usual after you eat Chinese food, try eating a little less rice, order a black bean side dish, and supplement your dinner with a high-soluble-fiber snack (see recipe in chapter 8). If your blood sugar tends to rise after having pasta, try eating a little less pasta next time and enjoy a salad loaded with kidney beans. See if it makes a difference.

When increasing the fiber in your diet, do so gradually and remember to drink a lot of sugar-free liquid along with high-fiber meals. More fluids will help reduce side effects common for an increase in fiber, such as diarrhea, flatulence, bloating, and abdominal pain. In most people, these side effects are temporary and disappear within a week or two of a continuous high-fiber diet.

CONSIDERING CALORIES

It's helpful to have a ballpark figure of how many calories you tend to eat and how many calories you should be shooting for, especially if you are a Type II whose diabetes may improve with some weight loss. That is not to say that everyone should be counting calories every day—once in a while will probably suffice. Your health care team might give you a target number of calories based on your age, sex, exercise habits, and the amount of calories you usually eat.

Knowing how closely you have been meeting this target number helps your health care team put all the pieces together. It helps them understand why you have or haven't lost some pounds. They can also calculate your target number of carbohydrate grams by calculating your target number of calories and working backward. Once you have your estimated daily calories, work with your dietitian to determine your desired percent of calories from carbohydrate. This might be 50 percent or 60 percent, or lower than 50 percent!

Divide this percentage by 100 to get .50 or .60, for example. Now you can multiply your daily calorie target by .50 or .60 to get the target *calories* from carbohydrate. Divide this number by 4 to get the target daily *grams* of carbohydrate. I've already calculated grams of carbohydrate for several calorie levels in the table on page 80.

Daily C-F-F Targets

We've already talked about how 30 grams of fiber a day is a fairly good target for those with diabetes, as well as for the average person. But the daily targets for carbohydrate grams and fat grams are not that straightforward. These numbers depend on your personal calorie needs, blood glucose management, and chronic disease risk factors such as obesity, high blood lipids, and so on.

We've discussed how some people with diabetes could manage their glucose well with a high-carbohydrate, low-fat eating plan, such as 60 percent calories from carbohydrate and 25 percent calories from fat. While others might manage well on a higher-fat, lower-carbohydrate eating plan, such as 45 percent calories from carbohydrate and 40 percent calories from fat (mostly monounsaturated fat). Even if you select your percentage of calories from one of the suggested carbohydrate and fat targets, the actual target of grams of carbohydrate and fat will vary from individual to individual, because each person consumes a different number of calories.

You may have already been given a carbohydrate target to work with by your health care team, or you may never have heard of carbo counting until this chapter. One of my friends, who is a normal weight Type II not on insulin, was given a target of carbohydrate grams by his dietitian for three meals, plus afternoon and evening snacks. My father, on the other hand, who is a Type II on mass quantities of insulin, was simply handed the exchange system when he was first diagnosed many years ago.

You can use the following table to help you estimate what your target grams of carbohydrate and fat might be, given a certain number of calories and the percentages you are striving to achieve from carbohydrate and from fat. For example, if you normally consume around 1,800 calories and you are

Target Grams of Carbohydrate and Fat

Daily Calories	Carbohydrate (g)			Fat (g)		
	If 40%	If 50%	If 60%	If 25%	If 35%	If 40%
	calories from carbohydrate			calories from fat		
1,200	120	150	180	33	47	53
1,500	150	188	225	42	58	67
1,800	180	225	270	50	70	80
2,100	210	263	315	58	82	93
2,400	240	300	360	67	93	107

trying the higher-carbohydrate (50 or 60 percent), lower-fat game plan, you might use 270 grams carbohydrate a day as your target. Make sure to go over this with your dietitian or certified diabetes educator before changing any previous eating plan.

CARBO-COUNTING WHEN ON INSULIN

You can also estimate your carbohydrate gram target amount by looking at how much insulin you are already taking and working backward. Most people need 1 unit of Regular (R) insulin (short-acting) or Humalog (rapid-acting) for each 10 to 15 grams of carbohydrate. This is called a carbohydrate-to-insulin ratio. And guess what? It varies from individual to individual. One person's carbohydrate-to-insulin ratio could be as high as 30 grams of carbohydrate per unit of insulin, to as low as 5 grams per unit of insulin. But *most* people fall in the 10 to 15 grams of carbohydrate per unit of insulin ratio. So if someone is taking 4 units of Regular (R) insulin in the morning, he might manage his blood sugar well on a 40-gram carbohydrate breakfast (4 × 10) or a 60-gram (4 × 15) carbohydrate breakfast. You'll need to work closely with your dietitian or certified diabetes educator to determine your carbohydrate-to-insulin ratio and to translate it into carbohydrate gram targets for each meal.

How to Find Your Carbohydrate-to-Insulin Ratio

Before you can determine your carbohydrate-to-insulin ratio and use it, you need to master three things—all of which entail receiving individual instructions and assistance from your health care team.

1. Your blood glucose levels should be under good control and the basal (NPH, Lente, ultraLente) dose of insulin well adjusted. Your basal insulin is the insulin that covers your nonfood insulin needs. Your insulin dose for each meal should be fine-tuned so that your blood glucose levels are within your target range before and after the meal. Your premeal target range may be 70 to 150 mg/dl, and your $1^1/_2$ to 2 hour postmeal target may be your premeal target plus 40 points but less than 180 mg/dl.
2. You have learned how to adjust your insulin based on patterns seen over several days of blood glucose records.
3. You have also learned how to use insulin supplements to correct blood glucose levels outside your target range. For example, you may have been advised to take 1 unit of Regular or Humalog insulin for each 50 points of blood glucose above your target. Or you may subtract insulin from your dose if your blood glucose is below your target.

You and your dietitian or certified diabetes educator can now review at least two weeks of records listing the carbohydrates you've eaten and the units of short-acting or rapid-acting insulin you've taken to meet your target blood glucose. The more insulin you require to cover your food, the lower the carbohydrate-to-insulin ratio will be. Many people can tolerate less carbohydrate per amount of insulin at breakfast than they can later in the day. For example, someone's breakfast ratio might be 10 grams carbohydrate per unit of insulin, while the dinner ratio is 15 to 1. Early-morning hormones make many people with diabetes less sensitive (more resistant) to insulin, causing high blood glucose and a need for more insulin in the morning.

A Word of Warning

If you do not know how much more (or less) insulin you need when your blood glucose is out of your target range, you will *not* get the best results possible, and you could also increase your risk of having severe hypoglycemia. Any experimenting with different doses and different amounts of carbohydrate should be done with the support of a health care team experienced in intensive insulin therapy and diabetes self-management.

This Is How It Works

First figure your dose of insulin based on the amount of carbohydrate that you plan to eat.

Then add or subtract the amount of insulin needed to bring your blood glucose into the target range. For example, suppose your premeal blood glucose is 200, your target range is 70 to 150, and you usually take 1 unit for each 50 points over 150 mg/dl. You will need to add 1 unit of Regular or Humalog insulin (200 actual − 150 target = 50 over) to correct for the higher premeal blood glucose. And if you plan to eat 60 grams of carbohydrate, and your ratio is 15 grams of carbohydrate per unit of insulin, you will need to take 4 units of insulin (60 divided by 15) to cover this carbohydrate: 4 + 1 = 5 total units of short-acting or rapid-acting insulin needed.

Unfortunately, after you have gone to all the trouble to find your carbohydrate-to-insulin ratio, you may have to do it again . . . and again. Weight gain usually increases your insulin requirements. Pregnancy, certain medications, and regular exercise may change your ratio as well.

What about Between-Meal Snacks?

Is your blood glucose low? If so, you may be advised not to take any insulin to cover the snack.

If you are eating a snack of less than 15 grams of carbohydrate within 2 to 3 hours of injecting mealtime insulin, you may not need an additional injection.

If you are planning to eat a snack of over 15 grams of carbohydrate within two to three hours of a mealtime insulin injection, you can figure the amount of insulin needed to cover the snack based on your carbohydrate-to-insulin ratio. If snack time is close to bedtime and you normally take NPH or Lente insulin at supper or bedtime, your health care team may advise you *not* to take any extra insulin to cover the snack.

Following Your Meal Plan Is Still Important

For Type IIs on insulin, it is still important to try to closely follow the meal plan your health care team has worked out with you. It is nice to have these insulin adjustment options for the occasional celebration dinner, but consuming more carbohydrate than estimated in your meal plan day after day can lead you toward weight gain.

Studies also show that following a meal plan consistently is linked with overall improved blood glucose control.

COMBINATION FOODS

Probably the biggest carbohydrate or C-F-F counting challenge is mixed foods. How do you count the carbohydrates, fat, and fiber in combinations of foods like potato and pasta salads, pizza, casseroles, lasagna, or sandwiches without a handy nutritional label? Do you pick the vegetables or meat off your pizza to measure them? Do you separate the noodles from the meat and gravy in a casserole? I tried to list as many combination foods as I could in the table on page 85 that concludes this chapter. This list is always here to help you count, but it is only an average value found in a particular food database. The most accurate way to count carbohydrates, fat, and fiber would be to separate the different components into groups and then measure them. This can be a little messy and time-consuming. I can just picture you with your sleeves rolled up, separating peas from rice.

Another way to go, especially if this is a recipe you or your spouse often make at home, is to computer-analyze the recipe and determine how much would be in each typical serving of that recipe. If you don't have access to a computer, you can look up the individual ingredients of the recipe using the table on page 85. You might have to add the numbers for noodles, chicken, vegetables, and gravy in a chicken noodle casserole, for example. Once you've done it, file the information right on your recipe card or keep a note card on the refrigerator with the information for your favorite recipes. If you would like me to analyze nutrients in your favorite recipes, follow the directions on my web page: www.recipemd.com.

BE YOUR OWN BLOOD GLUCOSE DETECTIVE I

It is really helpful to you and to your dietitian if you write down the foods you eat, how much, and when—along with any diabetes medication taken, physical activity, and blood glucose levels for about two weeks. Now you have ample clues to detect possible patterns in your blood glucose management. You must look especially carefully in three areas: medication, food, or exercise. These are three pieces of the blood glucose puzzle.

After going over your records with your dietitian or certified diabetes educator, you might need to adjust the amount or timing of exercise, your

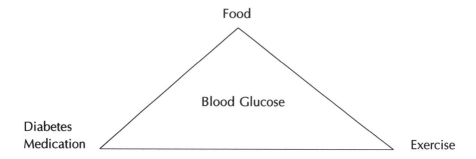

dose or timing of medication, or the amount or timing of carbohydrates in your meal plan. You might even want to try switching to lower glycemic-index carbohydrate foods like pasta, beans, or strawberries (foods that tend to raise the blood sugar *less* than higher glycemic-index foods) and/or boosting the soluble fiber total of certain meals.

Step 1: Look for blood glucose levels above and below your target ranges. (Your premeal blood glucose target range might be 70 to 120 or 150.) Are there patterns that repeat in your blood glucose records?

Step 2: Look for possible reasons why your blood glucose level was out-of-range each particular time.
- Did you have more or less carbohydrate at the previous meal or snack?
- Were you more or less active than usual?
- Was the previous meal particularly high or low in fat?
- Was the previous meal unusually high or low in fiber, particularly soluble fiber?
- Were you ill or under a lot of stress?
- Did you take your diabetes medication as directed? If so, perhaps your medication needs to be adjusted; ask your doctor or diabetes educator.

For example, if your blood glucose levels are too high before lunch, try circling the breakfasts where you ate more than 35 grams of carbohydrate. Are those the days when your prelunch blood glucose was high?

C-F-F counting is an ongoing mental exercise that no doubt will seem tiresome some days. Try to think of it as a challenge (I know, easy for me to say), which when met can improve your control over your life. Remember the attitude adjustment that makes the strategies in chapter 4 work.

I've tried to give you the information you'll need to succeed. Much more help is coming in the next three chapters.

Calculating C-F-F

Use this table to help count carbohydrate, fat, and fiber grams for a meal you are eating or planning to eat. You can also use it to help compute calories and grams of carbohydrate, fat, and fiber for days past. These totals are helpful for you and your health care team as a frame of reference, along with blood glucose records and information on physical activity.

	Calories	Carbo-hydrate (g)	Fat (g)	Fiber (g)	Sodium (mg)
Breads and Cereals					
Breads					
bagel, plain, 1 (2.5 oz.)	195	38.0	1.0	1.5	379
bagel, whole wheat, 1 (2 oz.)	145	31.0	1.0	5.5	228
bagel, cinnamon raisin, 1 (2.5 oz.)	194	39.0	1.0	2.0	228
bread crumbs, seasoned, 1 oz.	101	19.0	1.5	1.0	709
bun, hamburger, 1	129	22.5	1.0	0	252
bun, hot dog, 1	114	20.0	2.0	1.0	224
dinner roll, French, 1	105	19.0	1.5	1.0	231
English muffin, 1	134	26.0	1.0	1.5	265
French bread, 1 piece (1.25 oz.)	96	18.0	1.0	1.0	213
pita bread, 1 (2 oz.)	165	33.5	1.0	1.0	321
pumpernickel bread, 1 piece (1 oz.)	80	15.0	1.0	2.5	214
raisin bread, 1 piece (1 oz.)	69	13.0	1.0	1.0	98
sourdough bread, 1 piece (1 oz.)	69	13.0	1.0	1.0	152
white bread, 1 piece (1 oz.)	91	17.0	1.3	1.0	163
whole wheat bread, 1 piece (1.25 oz.)	86	16.0	1.5	2.0	184
Quick Breads					
cornbread, 1 piece (2.25 oz.)	176	28.0	5.0	2.0	427
date-nut bread, 1 piece (2 oz.)	216	30.0	10.0	1.0	140
Cold Cereal					
All Bran, 1/2 cup	107	32.0	0.8	15.0	486
Apple Jacks, 1 cup	110	25.5	0	0.5	125
Bran Buds, 1/2 cup	111	32.5	1.0	16.0	265
Bran Chex, 1/2 cup	78	19.5	0.7	4.0	227
bran flakes, 1 cup	127	30.5	0.7	5.5	303
Cap'n Crunch, 1 cup	156	30.0	3.4	0.7	278
Cheerios, 1 cup	89	15.7	1.5	1.6	246

(continued)

	Calories	Carbo-hydrate (g)	Fat (g)	Fiber (g)	Sodium (mg)
Cheerios, Honey Nut, 1 cup	125	26.5	0.8	1.5	299
corn flakes, 1 cup	97	21.5	0	0.7	256
Crispix, 1 cup	110	25.0	0	1.0	240
Frosted Flakes, 1 cup	144	34.0	0	0.7	306
Golden Grahams, 1 cup	150	33.0	1.5	1.4	386
Grape-Nuts, 1/2 cup	195	44.7	0.2	5.5	379
Kix, 1 cup	74	15.6	0.4	0.3	193
Life, 1 cup	163	31.5	0.8	2.6	230
Mueslix Five Grain Cereal, 1/2 cup	140	31.5	1.6	3.7	54
Nature Valley Granola, 1/2 cup	251	37.8	9.8	3.0	116
Post Alpha Bits, 1 cup	130	27.0	1.0	1.0	210
Product 19, 1 cup	126	27.4	0.2	1.4	378
Raisin Bran, 1/2 cup	87	21.0	0.6	3.0	155
Rice Chex, 1 cup	99	22.4	0	0.5	210
Rice Krispies, 1 cup	111	25.0	0	0	206
Shredded Wheat, 1/2 cup sm. biscuits	77	17.0	0.5	2.0	2
Special K, 1 cup	110	21.3	0	0.7	265
Total Wheat, 1 cup	116	26.0	0.7	4.3	326
Wheat Chex, 1/2 cup	85	19.0	0.6	2.0	154
Wheaties, 1 cup	101	23.0	0.5	2.6	276

Hot Cereal

	Calories	Carbo-hydrate (g)	Fat (g)	Fiber (g)	Sodium (mg)
Oatmeal, 1 cup, no salt added	145	25.3	2.3	4.0	2

Pastry

	Calories	Carbo-hydrate (g)	Fat (g)	Fiber (g)	Sodium (mg)
fruit-filled Danish, 1 (3.25 oz.)	335	45.0	16.0	N/A*	333
cheese Danish, 1 (2.25 oz.)	226	24.5	11.0	1.0	226
cake doughnut, 1 (1.8 oz.)	211	25.0	11.4	0.9	273
chocolate doughnut w/icing (2.5 oz.)	272	30.3	16.0	2.5	129
jelly-filled doughnut, 1 (2.25 oz.)	221	25.4	12.0	0.7	190
Pop-Tart, fruit filled, 1	212	37.0	5.5	0.7	226
raised doughnut, 1 (2 oz.)	241	26.6	13.7	1.3	205

Grains

Pasta (1/2 cup serving, cooked)

	Calories	Carbo-hydrate (g)	Fat (g)	Fiber (g)	Sodium (mg)
rotini	99	19.8	0.5	1.0	1
small shells	81	16.2	0.4	1.0	1

*Information not available.

	Calories	Carbo-hydrate (g)	Fat (g)	Fiber (g)	Sodium (mg)
macaroni, whole wheat	87	18.5	0.4	2.5	2
vermicelli	99	19.8	0.5	1.0	1
spaghetti	99	19.8	0.5	1.0	1

Rice ($^{1}/_{2}$ cup serving, cooked)

	Calories	Carbo-hydrate (g)	Fat (g)	Fiber (g)	Sodium (mg)
brown rice	108	22.5	0.9	1.8	5
white rice	133	29.0	0.3	0.6	1
white rice, instant	81	17.5	0.3	0.5	2
wild rice	83	17.5	0.3	1.0	2
flavored rice and pasta (Rice-A-Roni)	133	23.4	3.0	4.3	619
fried rice, meatless	130	17.0	5.8	0.7	141
Spanish rice	108	20.6	1.9	2.0	335

Beans ($^{1}/_{2}$ cup serving, unless noted otherwise)

	Calories	Carbo-hydrate (g)	Fat (g)	Fiber (g)	Sodium (mg)
baby lima beans, boiled	115	20.0	0.3	4.5	15
baked beans, homemade	190	27.0	6.5	7.0	531
baked beans, vegetarian	118	26.0	0.6	6.4	504
black beans, cooked with salt	114	20.4	0.5	8.0	204
broad beans/fava beans, canned	94	16.0	0.3	4.5	580
garbanzo beans, canned	143	27.0	1.4	4.5	359
Great Northern beans, cooked without salt	104	18.6	0.4	5.0	2
kidney beans, boiled	112	20.0	0.4	7.0	2
lima beans, canned	82	15.6	0.3	3.6	201
navy beans, cooked without salt	129	24.0	0.5	8.0	1
pink beans, boiled	125	23.4	0.4	4.5	2
pinto beans, cooked without salt	117	22.0	0.4	7.4	2
pork and beans, canned	124	24.5	1.3	6.1	557
refried beans, canned	135	23.4	1.4	6.7	537
white beans, boiled	127	22.6	0.6	5.7	2

Cheese and Dairy

Cheese

	Calories	Carbo-hydrate (g)	Fat (g)	Fiber (g)	Sodium (mg)
American, 1 slice (.75 oz.)	79	0.3	6.6	0	300
blue (.5 oz.)	50	0.3	4.0	0	198
brie (1 oz.)	95	0.1	8.0	0	178
cheddar (1 oz.)	114	0.4	9.4	0	176
cheddar, reduced fat (1 oz.)	90	<1	9.4	0	240

(continued)

	Calories	Carbo-hydrate (g)	Fat (g)	Fiber (g)	Sodium (mg)
Cheez Whiz (1 oz.)	82	2.5	6.0	0	381
feta (1 oz.)	75	1.0	6.0	0	316
gorganzola (1 oz.)	111	0	9.0	0	512
Gouda (1 oz.)	101	0.6	7.8	0	232
Monterey jack (1 oz.)	106	0.2	8.6	0	152
Monterey jack, reduced fat (1 oz.)	70	<1	4.5	0	200
mozzarella, low-fat (1 oz.)	79	0.8	5.0	0	150
Parmesan, 1/4 cup grated	114	1.0	7.5	0	465
provolone (1 oz.)	100	0.6	7.5	0	248
string, 1 stick (1 oz.)	72	0.8	4.5	0	132
Swiss (1 oz.)	107	1.0	7.8	0	74
Swiss, reduced fat (1 oz.)	51	1.0	1.5	0	74

Dairy

Milk

whole milk, 8 oz.	140	10.6	7.6	0	120
2% milk, 8 oz.	112	11.0	4.4	0	122
1% lowfat milk, 8 oz.	95	11.0	2.4	0	123
nonfat (skim) milk, 8 oz.	79	11.0	0.4	0	126
buttermilk, 8 oz.	92	11.0	2.2	0	257
evaporated skim milk, 4 oz.	99	13.0	0.3	0	147
evaporated whole milk, 4 oz.	169	11.5	9.5	0	134
chocolate milk, whole, 8 oz.	209	23.5	9.5	0	149
2% lowfat chocolate milk, 8 oz.	179	23.5	5.0	0	151

Cream

half-and-half, 1 Tb.	20	0.7	1.7	0	6
whipping, 2 Tb.	103	1.0	11.0	0	11
creamer, powder, 1 tsp.	11	1.0	0.7	0	4
nondairy creamer, 1 tsp.	10	1.0	0.5	0	5
whipped cream, pressurized, 1/2 cup	77	3.8	6.7	0	39
whipping cream, heavy, 1/2 cup whipped	205	1.7	22.0	0	21

Other Dairy

creamed cottage cheese, 1/2 cup	108	3.0	4.8	0	425
2% cottage cheese, 1/2 cup	101	4.0	2.0	0	459
1% cottage cheese, 1/2 cup	82	3.0	1.2	0	370
nonfat cottage cheese, 4 oz.	80	4.0	0	0	370
cottage cheese, low sodium-low fat, 1/2 cup	81	3.0	7.0	0	15
cream cheese, 1 oz.	99	1.0	10.0	0	84

	Calories	Carbo-hydrate (g)	Fat (g)	Fiber (g)	Sodium (mg)
light Neufchatel cheese, 1 oz.	81	3.0	7.0	0	117
cream cheese, light, 1 oz.	62	2.0	4.4	0	133
cream cheese, nonfat, 1 oz.	26	2.0	0	0	137
ricotta cheese, part skim, 1/2 cup	170	6.4	9.7	0	154
sour cream, 2 Tb.	62	1.0	6.0	0	15
light sour cream, 2 Tb.	41	2.0	2.5	0	20
imitation sour cream, 2 Tb.	60	2.0	5.6	0	29

Desserts

Cake (1-piece serving, unless noted otherwise)

	Calories	Carbo-hydrate (g)	Fat (g)	Fiber (g)	Sodium (mg)
angel food cake (1.9 oz.)	137	30.6	0.4	.8	397
applesauce cake with nuts and icing (4 oz.)	399	70.0	13.3	1.5	293
banana cake with icing (4 oz.)	309	58.5	7.6	1.1	292
carrot cake with cream cheese icing (4 oz.)	488	53.0	30.0	1.3	276
cheesecake (1/12 of 9-in. cake, 3.25 oz.)	295	23.5	21.0	2.0	190
chocolate cake with chocolate icing (2.5 oz.)	253	38.0	11.0	2.0	230
coffee cake, cinnamon (2 oz.)	240	30.0	12.0	1.0	233
coffee cake, cheese (2.7 oz.)	258	34.0	11.6	1.0	258
fruitcake (1.5 oz.)	155	28.0	5.0	1.6	62
German chocolate cake with icing (4 oz.)	404	55.0	21.0	1.6	369
lemon cake with icing, two layers (3.8 oz.)	388	70.3	11.3	0.5	248
pineapple upside down cake (4 oz.)	367	58.0	14.0	1.0	367
poppyseed cake, no icing (3.25 oz.)	354	43.0	17.5	1.0	251
pound cake, with butter (1 oz.)	113	14.0	5.8	0.2	115
sponge cake (2.25 oz.)	187	40.0	2.7	0.5	144
white cake with white icing (2.5 oz.)	266	44.5	9.6	0.7	166
yellow cake with chocolate icing (2.5 oz.)	262	38.2	12.0	1.2	233

Cookies

	Calories	Carbo-hydrate (g)	Fat (g)	Fiber (g)	Sodium (mg)
animal crackers/cookies, 5	51	8.4	1.6	N/A*	45
butter, 1	23	3.4	1.0	0.1	18

*Information not available.

(continued)

	Calories	Carbo-hydrate (g)	Fat (g)	Fiber (g)	Sodium (mg)
chocolate sandwich, creme-filled, 1	47	7.0	2.0	0.3	61
chocolate chip, small, soft, 1 (10.5 g)	49	6.0	3.0	0.3	36
fig bar, 1	49	10.0	1.0	0.6	49
Fig Newton, fat-free, 1	68	15.6	0	N/A	76
fudge cookie—cake type, 1 (21 g)	73	16.4	0.8	N/A	40
fortune, 1	30	6.7	0.2	0.1	22
gingersnap, 1	29	5.4	0.7	0.1	22
macaroon, 1	97	17.3	3.0	0.8	59
oatmeal raisin, 1 (13 g)	57	9.0	3.0	0.4	70
peanut butter, homemade, 1 (12 g)	57	7.0	3.0	0.2	62
Pecan Sandies, 1	75	9.8	3.5	0.3	9
shortbread, 1	40	5.0	2.0	0.1	37
snickerdoodle, 1 (.75 oz.)	81	11.7	3.5	0.4	68
vanilla wafer, 4 (.5 oz.)	70	11.8	2.4	N/A*	50
Frozen Yogurt (¹/₂ cup serving)					
nonfat chocolate	104	21.4	0.8	1.5	62
nonfat vanilla-fruit	96	19.0	0.2	0	65
soft-serve vanilla	114	17.4	4.0	0	63
low-fat chocolate	110	21.0	2.0	1.5	57
Ice Cream (¹/₂ cup serving)					
chocolate	178	24.0	8.4	0.7	44
strawberry	130	18.0	6.0	0.1	40
vanilla	133	15.6	7.3	0.1	53
soft-serve, vanilla	185	19.0	11.2	0.1	53
ice cream cookie sandwich (Chipwich), 1	144	21.8	5.6	0.6	36
Pie (¹/₈ of 9-in.-diameter pie, unless otherwise noted)					
apple	301	42.0	14.2	2.0	239
banana cream	399	49.0	20.0	N/A	356
black bottom	277	28.0	17.0	1.0	157
blackberry	402	56.0	19.0	4.5	294
blueberry	358	49.0	17.4	2.0	271
cherry	337	48.0	15.2	2.0	238
chocolate cream	399	44.0	23.0	N/A	347
coconut cream	433	50.0	23.0	N/A	390
custard (1/8 of 8-in.-diameter pie)	166	16.4	9.2	1.0	190
grasshopper	331	33.0	18.0	0.4	476
lemon meringue	362	49.5	16.4	N/A*	307

*Information not available.

	Calories	Carbo-hydrate (g)	Fat (g)	Fiber (g)	Sodium (mg)
pecan	503	63.5	27.0	N/A	320
pumpkin	303	39.0	13.8	N/A	335
sweet potato	307	34.0	16.4	1.7	190

Popsicles

popsicle/ice, double pops	92	24.0	0	0	15
vanilla pudding pop, 1	75	12.5	2.0	0	50

Pudding

bread, with raisins, 1 oz.	113	14.0	5.8	0.2	115
chocolate, homemade, with milk, ½ cup	221	40.3	5.7	1.3	137
instant chocolate, with 2% milk, ½ cup	150	21.8	2.8	1.0	417
rice, from mix, with 2% milk, ½ cup	161	30.2	2.3	0.3	158
tapioca, homemade, with milk, ½ cup	147	27.8	2.4	N/A	172
vanilla, with 2% milk, ½ cup	148	28.0	2.4	0.1	406
low-calorie (D-Zerta), with milk, ½ cup	88	12.0	2.4	0	303

Eggs and Egg Dishes

egg yolk, 1 large	60	0.3	5.0	0	7
egg white, 1 large	17	0.3	0	0	55
fried egg in margarine, 1 large	92	0.6	7.0	0	163
poached egg, 1 large	75	0.6	5.3	0	62
deviled egg (½ egg and filling)	62	0.4	5.0	0	94
scrambled egg with milk and margarine, 1 large	101	1.4	7.4	0	171
nonfat egg substitute, ¼ cup	30	1.0	0	0	100
quiche Lorraine, ⅛ of 9-in. diameter pie	508	20.0	39.0	0.6	550
omelet, with 1 large egg	90	0.6	6.8	0	160
omelet, with cheese and ham, 1 large egg	142	1.0	10.8	0	369
omelet, Spanish, 1 large egg	123	7.0	8.8	1.6	251
omelet, with sausage and mushrooms, 1 large egg	173	1.3	13.5	0.2	455

(continued)

	Calories	Carbo-hydrate (g)	Fat (g)	Fiber (g)	Sodium (mg)
Fats and Oils					
butter, 1 Tb.	102	0	11.5	0	117
butter, unsalted, 1 Tb.	102	0	11.5	0	2
Margarine					
hard margarine (stick), 1 Tb.	102	0	11.5	0	134
diet margarine (spread), 1 Tb.	49	0	5.5	0	50
Fleischmann's Light Margarine (tub), 1 Tb.	65	0	7.3	0	70
Touch of Butter Spread, 1 Tb.	53	0	6.0	0	70
Blue Bonnet Spread, 1 Tb.	102	0	11.5	0	127
liquid margarine, 1 Tb.	102	0	11.4	0	110
Oils					
olive oil, 1 Tb.	119	0	13.5	0	0
corn, safflower, soybean, canola oils, 1 Tb.	120	0	13.6	0	0
shortening, vegetable, 1 Tb.	113	0	12.8	0	0
Frozen Dinners					
Banquet					
Fried Chicken Dinner	470	35.0	27.0	6.0	960
Turkey Dinner	270	31.0	10.0	3.0	1100
Meatloaf Dinner	280	23.0	17.0	4.0	1100
Healthy Choice					
Sweet & Sour Chicken Dinner	310	42.0	5.0	5.0	250
Glazed Chicken Entree	200	30.0	1.5	3.0	480
Honey Mustard Chicken	260	40.0	2.0	4.0	550
Breast of Turkey Dinner	280	40.0	3.0	7.0	460
Chicken Parmigiana Dinner	300	47.0	1.5	6.0	490
Fettucini Alfredo Entree	240	39.0	5.0	3.0	430
Cacciatore Chicken	260	36.0	3.0	6.0	510
Fiesta Chicken Fajitas	260	36.0	4.0	5.0	410
Beef Pepper Steak Oriental	250	34.0	4.0	3.0	470
Lean Cuisine					
Oriental Beef with Veggies & Rice	240	29.0	8.0	4.0	461
Chicken Enchiladas	220	29.0	6.0	4.0	390

	Calories	Carbo-hydrate (g)	Fat (g)	Fiber (g)	Sodium (mg)
Chicken Fettucini	270	33.0	6.0	2.0	580
Chicken Parmesan	220	22.0	5.0	5.0	530
Chicken Pie	320	39.0	10.0	3.0	590
Chicken and Vegetable	240	30.0	5.0	5.0	520
Roasted Turkey Breast	290	48.0	4.0	3.0	530
Spaghetti with Meat Sauce	290	45.0	6.0	4.0	550
Lasagna with Meat Sauce	270	34.0	6.0	5.0	560
Fettucini Alfredo	270	38.0	7.0	7.0	590
Cheese Ravioli	250	32.0	8.0	4.0	500
French Bread Pepperoni Pizza	330	46.0	7.0	4.0	590
Stouffer's Entree					
Beef Ravioli	370	43.0	14.0	5.0	680
Chicken a la King	320	43.0	10.0	3.0	750
Chicken Divan	210	10.0	10.0	1.0	570
Chicken Enchilada	370	45.0	14.0	3.0	970
Lasagna and Meat	360	34.0	13.0	5.0	780
French Bread Sausage Pepperoni Pizza	460	45.0	25.0	4.0	1130
Weight Watchers					
Beef Enchiladas Ranchero	190	18.0	5.0	**0.0**	500
Chicken Fettucini	280	25.0	9.0	2.0	590
Chicken Marsala	150	22.0	2.0	6.0	500
Chicken Parmesan	230	25.0	6.0	2.0	470
Fried Fillet of Fish	230	25.0	8.0	2.0	450
Lasagna with Meat Sauce	290	34.0	7.0	7.0	580

Fruits and Vegetables

Fruits

	Calories	Carbo-hydrate (g)	Fat (g)	Fiber (g)	Sodium (mg)
apple, 1 medium with peel (4.9 oz.)	81	21.0	0.5	3.0	0
apple slices, with peel, 1 cup	65	17.0	0.4	22.0	0
banana, 1 (4 oz.)	105	27.0	0.5	2.3	1
blackberries, 1/2 cup	38	9.0	0.3	3.0	0
boysenberries, 1/2 cup	38	8.0	0.3	2.6	0
blueberries, 1/2 cup	41	10.2	0.3	2.0	4
cantaloupe, 1/4 melon (4.5 oz.)	47	11.0	0.4	1.0	12
casaba melon, 1/8 melon (7 oz.)	51	12.0	0.2	1.0	24

(continued)

	Calories	Carbo-hydrate (g)	Fat (g)	Fiber (g)	Sodium (mg)
cherries, sweet, 1/2 cup	52	12.0	0.7	1.0	0
cranberries, 1/2 cup	23	6.0	0.1	1.6	0
grapes, 1/2 cup	57	14.0	0.5	0.5	2
grapefruit, 1/2 cup sections	37	9.3	0.1	1.5	0
honeydew, 1/10 melon (4.5 oz.)	45	12.0	0.1	1.0	13
kiwi fruit, 1	46	11.3	0.3	1.5	4
mandarin oranges, canned, 1/2 cup sections	47	12.0	0	0.4	6
melon balls (mixed), 1/2 cup	29	7.0	0.2	0.6	27
nectarine, 1 (5 oz.)	67	16.0	0.6	2.0	0
nectarine slices, 1/2 cup	34	8.0	0.3	1.0	0
orange, 1 medium (5 oz.)	62	15.5	0.3	1.0	0
peach, 1 medium (3 oz.)	37	10.0	0	1.6	0
peach slices, 1/2 cup	37	10.0	0	1.5	0
pear, 1 medium (6 oz.)	98	25.0	0.7	4.0	0
pear slices, 1/2 cup	49	12.0	0.3	2.0	0
pineapple chunks, fresh, 1/2 cup	38	9.6	0.3	1.0	1
plum, 1 medium (2.5 oz.)	36	8.6	0.4	1.3	0
raspberries, 1/2 cup	30	7.0	0.3	2.4	0
strawberries, whole, 1/2 cup	22	5.0	0.3	1.0	1
strawberries, 1/2 cup slices	25	6.0	0.3	1.3	1
watermelon, 1/2 cup chunks	26	5.8	0.3	0.2	2
watermelon, 1-by-10-in. slice	154	35.0	2.0	1.0	10

Fruit and Vegetable Juices

	Calories	Carbo-hydrate (g)	Fat (g)	Fiber (g)	Sodium (mg)
apple juice, bottled, 8 oz.	117	26.5	0.3	0.2	7
cranberry juice cocktail, 8 oz.	144	32.5	0.3	0.2	5
grape juice, bottled, 8 oz.	154	34.0	0.2	0.2	8
grapefruit juice, 8 oz.	88	21.0	0.2	0.2	2
orange juice, unsweetened, 8 oz.	112	23.5	0.4	0.5	2
pineapple juice, unsweetened, 8 oz.	140	31.3	0.2	0.2	3
prune juice, bottled, 8 oz.	182	40.0	0.1	2.3	10
tomato juice, low-sodium, canned, 8 oz.	42	9.6	0.1	1.8	880
vegetable juice (V-8), 8 oz.	46	9.5	0	1.4	884
vegetable juice (V-8), low sodium, 8 oz.)	46	10.3	0	1.8	60

Vegetables (1/2 cup serving, unless noted otherwise)

	Calories	Carbo-hydrate (g)	Fat (g)	Fiber (g)	Sodium (mg)
acorn squash, baked, mashed (4.25 oz.)	67	18.0	0.2	5.0	5

	Calories	Carbo-hydrate (g)	Fat (g)	Fiber (g)	Sodium (mg)
baby carrots, 5	19	4.0	0.3	1.6	18
beet greens, boiled	20	4.0	0.1	2.0	174
beet greens, raw, chopped	4	0.8	0	1.0	38
beets, boiled	37	8.5	0.1	1.5	65
broccoli, steamed	22	4.0	0.3	2.3	20
broccoli florets, raw	12	2.3	0.2	1.3	12
broccoli cooked with cheese sauce	111	6.3	7.3	2.0	365
broccoli cooked with cream sauce	93	7.1	5.8	2.0	345
Brussels sprouts, cooked	30	6.8	0.4	3.6	16
butternut squash, baked, mashed	49	13.0	0.1	3.4	5
cabbage, shredded, raw	9	2.0	0.1	0.7	6
cabbage, chopped, steamed	19	4.0	0.2	2.0	14
cabbage, cooked	17	3.4	0.3	2.0	4
carrot, 1 whole	31	7.3	0.1	1.9	25
carrots, raw, grated	24	5.5	0.1	1.4	19
carrot slices, steamed	34	8.0	0.1	2.3	27
celery, raw, chopped	10	2.0	0.1	1.0	52
celery, 1 large outer stalk	6	1.5	0	0.6	35
Chinese cabbage, steamed	11	2.0	0.2	0.9	55
collard greens, boiled	17	4.0	0.1	1.3	10
corn, fresh	66	14.5	0.9	2.0	12
corn-on-the-cob, 1 small (2.75 oz.)	72	17.2	0.6	2.5	3
crookneck squash, boiled	18	4.0	0.3	1.3	1
dandelion greens, boiled	17	3.4	0.3	1.5	23
dandelion greens, raw, chopped	12	2.5	0.2	1.0	21
green beans, boiled	22	5.0	0.2	2.0	2
green beans (Italian style), frozen, boiled	18	4.0	0.1	2.0	9
Hubbard squash, baked, mashed	60	1.3	0.7	3.2	10
kale, cooked	21	3.7	0.3	1.3	15
mushroom pieces, raw	9	1.6	0.1	0.5	1
mushroom pieces, canned	19	4.0	0.2	2.0	332
mustard greens, boiled	11	1.5	0.2	1.5	11
mustard greens, raw, chopped	7	1.4	0	0.5	7
parsnips, raw slices	50	12.0	0.2	3.3	7
parsnips, boiled	63	15.2	0.2	3.5	8
peas, frozen, boiled	62	11.3	0.2	4.4	70
snow peas, boiled	34	7.7	0.2	3.4	3
spaghetti squash, boiled	23	5.0	0.2	1.0	14

(continued)

	Calories	Carbo-hydrate (g)	Fat (g)	Fiber (g)	Sodium (mg)
spinach, boiled	27	5.0	0.2	2.4	82
spinach, raw, chopped	6	1.0	0.1	0.8	22
split peas, dry, boiled	116	20.7	0.4	3.4	2
squash slices, boiled	18	4.0	0.3	1.3	1
sweet potato, candied, 2 pieces	142	29.0	3.0	2.0	73
sweet potato, 1 medium, with skin	117	27.7	0.1	3.4	11
Swiss chard, cooked	18	3.6	0.1	1.8	156
tomato, sun-dried, 1 oz. oil-pack, drained	60	6.6	4.0	1.8	75
tomato, 1 medium, ripe	26	5.7	4.0	1.8	75
tomatoes, stewed, low sodium	33	8.2	0.4	1.3	11
tomatoes, green, chopped	22	4.6	0.2	1.4	12
tomatoes, fried green, 1 (5 oz.)	238	16.4	18.0	2.0	243
turnip cubes, raw	18	4.0	0.1	1.6	44
turnip cubes, boiled	14	3.8	0.1	1.5	39
turnip greens, boiled	14	3.1	0.2	2.2	21
turnip greens, raw, chopped	7	1.6	0.1	0.7	11
winter squash, baked, mashed	47	10.6	0.8	3.4	1
yams, orange, baked	103	24.3	0.1	3.0	10
zucchini, raw	9	1.9	0.1	1.0	2
zucchini, slices, steamed	14	2.6	0.1	1.0	3

Lettuce (1 cup serving, unless noted otherwise)

	Calories	Carbo-hydrate (g)	Fat (g)	Fiber (g)	Sodium (mg)
butterhead, chopped	4	0.6	0	0.4	1
iceberg/crisp head, chopped	4	0.6	0	0.3	3
looseleaf, chopped	5	1.0	0	0.4	3
Romaine, chopped	5	0.7	0	0.4	2

Potatoes

	Calories	Carbo-hydrate (g)	Fat (g)	Fiber (g)	Sodium (mg)
baked potato with skin, 1 long (7 oz.)	220	51.5	0.2	5.0	16
hash brown potatoes, 1/2 cup	119	5.8	10.8	1.5	19
hash browns, fast-food serving	136	13.5	8.3	1.4	262
mashed potatoes with milk and salt, 1/2 cup	81	18.5	0.6	2.0	318
Tater Tots, 1/2 cup	138	19.0	6.6	2.0	463
scalloped potatoes (from mix), 1/2 cup	105	13.2	4.5	1.3	411
French fries, frozen (2 oz.)	114	15.7	5.3	1.3	418

	Calories	Carbo-hydrate (g)	Fat (g)	Fiber (g)	Sodium (mg)
Meat and Poultry					
Meat					
Beef (3 oz. cooked serving, unless noted otherwise)					
bottom round, lean, braised	187	0	8.0	0	43
chuck roast, lean and fat, braised	282	0	20.0	0	51
corned beef, cooked, trimmed	213	0	16.2	0	964
eye of round, lean and fat, braised	195	0	11.0	0	50
filet mignon, broiled, trimmed	179	0	8.5	0	54
flank steak, broiled	176	0	8.6	0	71
ground beef, extra-lean, grilled	224	0	13.6	0	69
London broil, broiled, trimmed of visible fat	176	0	8.6	0	71
porterhouse, lean and fat, broiled	259	0	18.8	0	52
porterhouse, lean, broiled	185	0	9.2	0	56
pot roast, lean and fat, roasted	234	0	14.0	0	43
rib-eye steak, broiled, trimmed of visible fat	191	0	9.9	0	59
round eye, lean, roasted	149	0	4.9	0	53
round steak, lean and fat, roasted	205	0	12.0	0	50
rump roast, lean and fat, braised	220	0	12.0	0	43
short ribs, lean, braised	251	0	15.4	0	49
short ribs with sauce	255	0	20.6	0	356
sirloin steak, lean, broiled	172	0	6.8	0	56
stew meat, lean	199	0	9.6	0	253
tenderloin steak, lean, broiled	179	0	8.5	0	54
T-bone, lean and fat, broiled	253	0	18.0	0	52
T-bone, lean only, broiled	182	0	8.9	0	56
top round, lean, broiled	153	0	4.2	0	52
top sirloin, lean and fat, broiled	241	0	15.6	0	53
Lamb (4 oz. cooked serving, unless noted otherwise)					
loin chop with visible fat	357	0	26.2	0	87
loin chop, lean only	245	0	11.0	0	95
rib roast, with visible fat	407	0	33.8	0	83
rib roast, lean only	263	0	15.0	0	92

(continued)

	Calories	Carbo- hydrate (g)	Fat (g)	Fiber (g)	Sodium (mg)
leg of lamb, with visible fat	292	0	18.7	0	75
leg of lamb, lean only	216	0	8.8	0	77

Pork (4 oz. cooked serving, unless noted otherwise)

	Calories	Carbo- hydrate (g)	Fat (g)	Fiber (g)	Sodium (mg)
ham, whole, roasted, lean only	178	0	6.0	0	1504
loin chop, with visible fat, broiled	357	0	25.0	0	79
loin chop, lean only, broiled	309	0	16.6	0	85
loin center chop, lean only, broiled	261	0	12.0	0	89
shoulder, with visible fat, braised	391	0	29.0	0	100
center rib chop, with visible fat, roasted	360	0	26.7	0	50
center rib chop, broiled	277	0	15.7	0	52
spareribs, with visible fat, braised	450	0	34.3	0	105
spareribs, no visible fat, braised	266	0	15.4	0	71

Poultry (3 oz. cooked serving, unless noted otherwise)

	Calories	Carbo- hydrate (g)	Fat (g)	Fiber (g)	Sodium (mg)
chicken breast, roasted	168	0	6.6	0	60
skinless chicken breast, roasted	140	0	3.0	0	63
chicken breast, floured, fried with skin	189	1.4	7.6	0	65
skinless chicken breast, fried	159	0.4	4.0	0	67
chicken breast, roasted	140	0	3.0	0	63
chicken drumstick, floured, fried	208	1.4	12.0	0	77
chicken drumstick, roasted	184	0	9.5	0	77
chicken thigh, floured, fried with skin	223	2.7	12.8	0	75
chicken thigh, roasted	210	0	13.2	0	71
skinless chicken thigh, fried	185	0	9.0	0	81
skinless chicken thigh, roasted	178	0	9.3	0	75
chicken wing, floured, fried	273	2.0	19.0	0	66
chicken wing, roasted	247	0	16.6	0	70
fast-food chicken, 2 pieces, dark meat	430	0	26.6	0	754
fast-food chicken nuggets, 4 pieces	209	9.5	14.0	N/A*	445
turkey white meat, roasted	168	0	7.0	0	54
turkey dark meat, roasted	188	0	9.8	0	65

Lunch Meats and Meat Products (2 oz. serving, unless noted otherwise)

	Calories	Carbo- hydrate (g)	Fat (g)	Fiber (g)	Sodium (mg)
bacon, 2 pieces, cooked	220	0	18.8	0	610
bacon, turkey (Louis Rich), 2 pieces	60	0	5.0	0	380

*Information not available.

	Calories	Carbo-hydrate (g)	Fat (g)	Fiber (g)	Sodium (mg)
bacon (Sizzlean), 2 pieces	99	0	7.6	0	496
beef lunch meat, thinly sliced	100	0	2.2	0	817
bologna, beef	177	0	16.2	0	557
bologna, turkey	113	0	8.6	0	497
bologna (Healthy Favorites)	56	0	1.2	0	629
chicken or turkey breast, smoked	62	0	1.0	0	811
chicken breast, roasted, Deli Thin (Louis Rich)	65	0	1.6	0	676
frankfurter, 1 beef and pork	182	1.0	16.6	0	638
frankfurter, 1 turkey	102	1.0	8.0	0	642
frankfurter, 1 chicken	116	1.0	8.8	0	617
frankfurter (Healthy Favorites), 1	60	1.0	1.5	0	570
ham, regular	103	0	6.0	0	747
ham slices, extra lean	74	0	2.8	0	810
olive loaf	133	9.4	9.4	0	842
Polish sausage, pork	185	1.0	16.3	0	510
Polska kielbasa, turkey	80	1.2	4.5	0	510
roast beef, deli thin (Oscar Mayer)	65	0	1.6	0	578
salami, 50% less fat (Gallo), 5 slices (1 oz.)	60	1.5	1.0	0	520
salami, dry	237	1.5	19.5	0	1055
sausage links, pork, 2 (1 oz.)	96	0	8.0	0	336
sausage patties, pork, 2 (2 oz.)	199	0	16.8	0	698
turkey-ham, thigh	73	0	3.0	0	565

Mixed Dishes

	Calories	Carbo-hydrate (g)	Fat (g)	Fiber (g)	Sodium (mg)
burrito, chicken (Taco Bell), 1	345	41.0	13.0	N/A*	854
burrito, seven-layer (Taco Bell), 1	458	55.0	19.5	8.5	983
burrito, beef, 1 whole	262	29.0	10.4	1.0	746
burrito, bean, 1 whole	224	35.7	6.8	4.0	493
burrito supreme with red sauce (Taco Bell), 1	443	51.0	19.0	5.0	1184
chicken or turkey noodle casserole, 1/2 cup	163	14.0	6.4	1.0	366
chicken club sandwich (Wendy's), 1 whole	520	44.0	25.0	2.0	990
chicken fillet sandwich, 1	515	39.0	19.5	1.3	957
chicken sandwich with cheese, 1	632	41.5	38.8	N/A*	1238

*Information not available.

(continued)

	Calories	Carbo-hydrate (g)	Fat (g)	Fiber (g)	Sodium (mg)
broiled chicken breast sandwich (Burger King Broiler), 1 whole	540	41.0	29.0	2.0	480
corn dog, 1 whole	460	56.0	19.0	N/A	973
chicken corn dog, 1 whole	272	26.0	13.0	N/A	670
fajita, chicken, 1 (8 oz.)	405	50.0	13.0	4.4	439
fajita, beef, 1 (8 oz.)	409	46.0	17.5	3.8	850
Fish Supreme sandwich, 1 whole	590	51.0	32.0	0	1170
ham and cheese submarine (8 oz.)	530	31.0	34.0	3.5	1727
hamburger (Burger King "Whopper"), 1	630	45.0	39.0	0	742
hamburger with cheese (4 oz.)	510	39.0	27.0	0	1030
hamburger, 1 patty	310	29.0	13.0	0.3	580
hamburger, double with condiments, 1	576	39.0	32.5	N/A	742
hot dog, super size, 4 oz. (Dairy Queen), 1	590	41.0	38.0	N/A	1360
hot dog, chicken, on bun, 1	235	24.0	11.0	1.0	819
hot dog with bun, 1	280	23.0	16.0	0.3	700
hot dog with chili, 1	320	26.0	19.0	2.3	720
lasagna, meatless, 1 piece (8 oz.)	298	39.0	9.3	3.3	714
lasagna with meat, 1 piece	382	39.0	15.2	3.3	745
roast beef sandwich (Hardee's), 1 regular	270	28.0	11.0	N/A*	780
macaroni and cheese, 1/2 cup	215	8.0	11.0	0	543
spaghetti with meatballs, 1/2 cup	166	19.0	6.0	4.0	505
spaghetti with white clam sauce, 1/2 cup	229	21.0	10.0	2.0	218
spaghetti with red clam sauce, 1/2 cup	144	20.5	3.8	2.0	153
taco, beef, 1 large (6 oz.)	369	27.0	20.5	N/A	802
taco, soft, chicken, 1 (4.5 oz.)	223	20.0	10.0	N/A	553
taco salad, with salsa and shells (Taco Bell) (20.5 oz.)	940	70.0	60.0	11.0	1171
taco salad (18 oz.), 1	430	30.0	24.0	N/A	716
tostada, 1 bean and chicken	253	19.0	11.4	3.5	435
tostada, 1 beef and cheese	315	23.0	26.3	N/A	897
tuna noodle casserole, 1/2 cup	119	13.0	3.7	1.0	388
turkey sandwich, 1 whole (approx. 7 oz.)	260	33.0	6.0	0.5	1270
turkey submarine sandwich (10 oz.)	486	46.5	19.0	N/A	2030

*Information not available.

	Calories	Carbo-hydrate (g)	Fat (g)	Fiber (g)	Sodium (mg)
Nuts and Nut Products					
filberts/hazelnuts, 1/2 cup	426	10.5	42.2	5.0	2
peanuts, oil roasted, unsalted, 1/2 cup	419	14.0	35.5	4.5	4
peanuts, dry roasted, unsalted, 1/2 cup	427	16.0	36.0	5.0	4
macadamia nuts, 1/2 cup	471	9.0	49.0	3.6	3
pistachios, dry roasted, 1/2 cup	388	18.0	33.8	7.0	499
walnuts, black, 1/2 cup chopped	379	7.5	35.4	2.8	1
walnuts, English, 1/2 cup halves	321	9.0	31.0	2.3	5
pine nuts, 2 oz.	292	8.0	28.7	2.5	2
soy nuts, 1/2 cup	190	13.0	10.0	1.5	2
mixed nuts, dry roasted, unsalted, 1/2 cup	407	17.0	35.5	6.0	8
mixed nuts, dry roasted, 1/2 cup	407	17.0	35.5	6.0	458
water chestnuts, 1/2 cup canned	35	9.0	0	1.8	6
almond butter, unsalted, 2 Tb.	203	7.0	19.0	2.0	4
almond butter, salted, 2 Tb.	198	7.0	18.5	2.0	141
peanut butter, 2 Tb.	188	7.0	16.0	2.0	156
peanut butter, unsalted, 2 Tb.	188	7.0	16.0	2.0	5
sunflower seed butter, 2 Tb.	185	9.0	15.3	2.0	166
tahini (sesame butter), 2 Tb.	182	5.0	17.0	3.0	0

Salads (1/2 cup serving, unless noted otherwise)

	Calories	Carbo-hydrate (g)	Fat (g)	Fiber (g)	Sodium (mg)
potato salad with mayo and eggs	179	14.0	10.3	2.0	661
potato salad, no egg	134	16.0	7.2	2.0	337
German potato salad	79	14.5	1.6	1.5	201
macaroni salad, no cheese	227	13.0	18.8	2.0	181
macaroni salad, low fat	159	25.0	4.5	1.5	568
coleslaw	89	8.0	6.7	1.0	162
tossed green salad	12	2.5	0.2	1.0	7
shrimp salad	142	3.0	8.4	0.4	188
tuna salad	192	10.0	9.5	0.6	412
chicken salad with celery	268	1.0	24.7	0.2	201

(continued)

	Calories	Carbo-hydrate (g)	Fat (g)	Fiber (g)	Sodium (mg)
Seafood					
abalone, fried, 3 oz.	160	9.0	6.0	0.4	502
abalone, steamed or poached, 3 oz.	178	10.0	1.3	0	384
bluefish, baked or broiled, 4 oz.	180	0	6.2	0	87
bluefish, fried in crumbs, 4 oz.	232	12.0	11.0	0	76
crab, dungeness, steamed or boiled, 1/2 cup	65	0	0.7	0	223
crab, blue, canned, 1/2 cup	67	0	0.8	0	225
crab, imitation, 3 oz.	87	0	1.0	0	715
crab, snow, baked or broiled, 3 oz.	117	0	5.4	0	459
crab, soft-shell, breaded and fried, 3 oz.	284	15.0	17.0	0	439
crab cakes, 1 (2 oz.)	93	0.3	4.5	0	198
fish patty or square, 2 (4 oz.)	311	27.0	14.0	0.5	665
fish sandwich with tartar sauce, 1 (5 oz.)	431	41.0	22.7	0.4	615
fish sandwich with cheese and tartar sauce, 1 (6.5 oz.)	524	48.0	28.6	0.4	940
fish sticks, frozen and heated, 4 (4 oz.)	310	27.0	14.0	0.5	663
Gefiltefish, sweet, 4 oz.	95	8.0	2.0	0	594
lobster, baked or broiled, 1/2 cup	84	0	2.2	0	450
lobster tail, batter-fried, 3 oz.	180	7.0	9.4	0	327
lobster with butter sauce, 1/2 cup	224	0	17.7	1.0	451
oysters, Eastern, breaded and fried, 1/2 cup	129	7.5	8.3	0	273
oysters, canned, 1/2 cup	86	0	3.0	0	139
oysters, baked or broiled, 1/2 cup	62	0	1.6	0	210
Pacific rockfish, baked or broiled, 4 oz.	137	0	2.3	0	87
prawns or jumbo shrimp, steamed or broiled, 3 oz.	84	0	1.0	0	191
salmon, baked or broiled, 4 oz.	206	0	9.0	0	64
shrimp, small or medium, steamed or boiled, 3 oz.	84	0	9.0	0	191
shrimp or prawns, breaded and fried, 3 oz.	206	10.0	10.5	0	293
shrimp, battered and fried, 1/2 cup	158	7.5	8.0	0	295
squid, floured and fried, 1/2 cup	131	6.0	5.6	0.2	229

	Calories	Carbo-hydrate (g)	Fat (g)	Fiber (g)	Sodium (mg)
squid or calamari, baked, 1/2 cup	97	0	3.3	0	259
swordfish, baked or broiled, 4 oz.	176	0	5.8	0	130
whitefish, baked or broiled, 4 oz.	195	0	8.5	0	74

Snacks

Chips (1 oz. serving, unless noted otherwise)

corn chips	153	16.0	9.5	1.4	179
light potato chips	133	19.0	6.0	1.3	140
potato chips, sour cream & onion	151	14.5	9.6	1.5	177
potato chips	152	15.0	9.8	1.3	169
Pringles light chips	142	18.0	7.3	1.0	121
tortilla chips (Doritos)	141	18.0	7.3	2.0	201
light tortilla chips	126	20.5	4.3	2.0	284

Crackers

butter crackers (Club), 7 (1 oz.)	141	17.0	7.0	0.5	237
butter crackers (Ritz), 10 (1 oz.)	151	18.0	7.6	0.6	254
butter crackers, reduced fat, 10 (1 oz.)	140	20.0	5.0	0.6	280
cheese crackers (Cheez-It), 30	151	17.5	7.6	1.0	299
graham crackers, 4 (1 oz.)	118	21.5	3.0	1.0	169
matzo cracker, 1 (1 oz.)	112	23.5	0.4	1.0	1
Saltines, 10 (1 oz.)	130	21.5	3.5	1.0	391
100% Stoned Wheat, 8 (1 oz.)	129	22.0	4.4	3.0	172
wheat crackers (Wheat Thins), 10 (1 oz.)	143	19.0	6.7	1.7	261
Wasa Rye Crisp, 4 (1 oz.)	117	26.0	0.4	3.0	300
whole wheat cracker (Triscuits), 7 (1 oz.)	140	21.5	5.4	3.3	208

Granola Bars

hard granola bar, 1 (1 oz.)	134	18.0	5.6	1.5	84
soft granola bar, 1 (1 oz.)	126	19.0	4.9	1.3	79
peanut butter soft granola bar, chocolate coated, 1 (1.3 oz.)	187	19.5	11.4	1.0	71
chocolate chip soft granola bar, 1 (1.5 oz.)	179	29.5	7.0	2.0	116

(continued)

	Calories	Carbo-hydrate (g)	Fat (g)	Fiber (g)	Sodium (mg)
Fi-Bar, yogurt-coated granola bar, 1 (1 oz.)	107	18.5	3.0	2.2	5

Other

	Calories	Carbo-hydrate (g)	Fat (g)	Fiber (g)	Sodium (mg)
BBQ Corn nuts, 3 oz.	371	61.0	12.2	7.0	830
popcorn, air popped, 1 oz. (3½ cups)	108	22.0	1.2	4.2	1
popcorn, oil popped, salted, 1 oz. (2¾ cups)	142	17.5	8.0	3.0	251
caramel corn, 1 oz. (1 cup)	122	22.5	3.6	1.5	58

Soups and Canned Entrees (½ cup serving, unless noted otherwise)

	Calories	Carbo-hydrate (g)	Fat (g)	Fiber (g)	Sodium (mg)
bean and bacon soup with water	86	12.5	3.0	3.5	476
beef stew	97	8.7	3.8	1.2	503
birds nest soup (chicken, ham, noodles)	56	3.0	1.4	0	754
black bean soup with water	58	10.0	0.8	2.2	599
bouillabaisse soup/chowder	121	2.4	4.5	0.3	209
chicken gumbo soup with water	28	4.2	0.7	1.0	477
chicken noodle soup with water	37	4.7	1.2	0.4	553
chicken rice soup with water	30	3.6	1.0	0.4	408
chunky chicken noodle	88	11.0	3.0	1.0	425
chunky chicken rice soup	64	10.5	1.6	1.0	444
chunky chicken vegetable soup	59	6.5	1.7	0	378
chunky minestrone	64	10.5	1.4	1.0	432
chunky split pea & ham soup	93	13.0	2.0	1.5	483
chunky vegetable soup	61	9.5	1.9	0.6	505
chunky turkey soup	68	7.0	2.2	0.5	462
cream of broccoli soup	117	8.0	8.0	1.0	394
cream of chicken soup with milk	96	7.5	5.8	0	523
cream of chicken soup with water	58	4.5	3.7	0	493
cream of mushroom soup with milk	102	7.5	6.8	0.2	538
cream of mushroom soup with water	65	4.7	4.5	0.2	516
cream of potato soup with milk	75	8.5	3.0	0.3	531
cream of potato soup with water	37	6.0	1.2	0.3	500
chili, vegetarian	144	15.0	2.0	4.0	526
chili and beans	143	15.0	7.0	5.5	666
egg drop soup	37	0.6	2.0	0	365
gazpacho soup	28	0.4	1.0	1.8	590
lentil and ham soup	70	10.0	1.4	1.0	660

	Calories	Carbo- hydrate (g)	Fat (g)	Fiber (g)	Sodium (mg)
low sodium cream of mushroom soup	65	4.5	4.5	0.2	24
low sodium pea soup	83	13.0	1.5	0.4	13
low sodium vegetable soup	41	6.5	1.2	0.4	21
low sodium vegetable chicken soup	83	9.5	2.4	0.5	42
minestrone with water	41	5.5	1.3	0.5	456
mushroom barley soup with water	37	6.0	1.0	0.4	446
spaghetti sauce	136	20.0	6.0	4.0	618
spaghetti sauce with meatballs	128	14.0	5.0	1.0	553
split pea and ham soup with water	95	14.0	2.0	2.5	503
tomato beef noodle soup with water	70	10.5	2.2	1.0	459
tomato bisque soup with milk	99	14.5	3.3	0	555
tomato bisque soup with water	62	12.0	1.3	0	524
tomato rice soup with water	60	11.0	1.4	0.7	408
tomato soup with milk	81	11.0	3.0	0.2	466
tomato soup with water	43	8.0	1.0	0.2	436
vegetable soup with water	36	8.0	0.5	1.0	411
wonton soup	94	8.0	3.5	0.5	380

Candy

	Calories	Carbo- hydrate (g)	Fat (g)	Fiber (g)	Sodium (mg)
Butterfinger, 1 (2 oz.)	286	42.5	11.4	1.5	121
chocolate-covered peanuts, 1/2 cup (3 oz.)	441	42.0	28.5	3.5	35
Kit Kat, 1 (1.5 oz.)	214	26.0	12.0	0.4	42
milk chocolate candy bar, 1 (1.5 oz.)	226	26.0	13.5	1.5	36
3 Musketeers, 1 (2 oz.)	251	46.0	7.8	1.0	117

Beverages

Alcohol

	Calories	Carbo- hydrate (g)	Fat (g)	Fiber (g)	Sodium (mg)
beer (12 oz.)	146	12.5	0	0	18
beer, light (12 oz.)	99	4.5	0	0	11
gin, whiskey, brandy, rum, vodka (1 oz.)	75	0	0	0	1
wine, red (6 oz.)	127	3.0	0	0	9
wine, white (6 oz.)	120	1.0	0	0	9

(continued)

	Calories	Carbo- hydrate (g)	Fat (g)	Fiber (g)	Sodium (mg)
Cocoa					
hot chocolate with whole milk, 3/4 cup (6 oz.)	164	19.0	7.0	2.0	92
hot chocolate mix plus water, 1 packet (3/4 cup)	103	21.0	1.0	2.0	148
Soda (12 oz. serving)					
cola	152	35.0	0	0	15
cola, caffeine free	153	35.0	0	0	24
diet cola, caffeine free	0	0	0	0	51
7-Up	151	35.0	0	0	10
Slice	156	35.0	0	0	15
diet Slice type	7	0.3	0	0	1
ginger ale	115	29.5	0	0	26
root beer	152	36.0	0	0	48
cream soda	189	45.0	0	0	45
orange soda	179	42.0	0	0	45
grape soda	160	38.0	0	0	56
Other					
fruit punch, canned (8 oz.)	119	27.0	0	0	56
fruit punch, low-calorie (8 oz.)	43	11.0	0	0	50
cappuccino coffee mix plus water (6 oz.)	61	10.0	2.0	0	104
Swiss mocha coffee mix plus water (6 oz.)	50	7.5	2.0	0	36

6

ALL THE ADVICE AND DATA YOU NEED TO MANAGE YOUR DIET

I know I've thrown a lot of numbers at you in the process of discussing dietary goals and theories. Now we get to the real hands-on stuff, what you need to do to achieve the control you want. Just in case all the dietary data and advice have become a bit muddled, let's review briefly.

There is some individual variation on dietary management of diabetes, but in most cases people are encouraged to eat:

- around 10 to 20 percent of calories from protein (combination animal and vegetable proteins)
- less than 10 percent of calories from saturated fat (Americans consume about 13 percent of daily calories from saturated fat)
- up to 10 percent of calories from polyunsaturated fat
- 60 to 70 percent of calories from a combination of carbohydrates and monounsaturated fat
- about 30 to 40 grams of fiber a day (or 15 to 25 grams per 1,000 calories) from both soluble and insoluble fibers (American men typically take in 19 grams a day while women take in about 13.)
- enough calories to achieve a more healthful body weight

Some experts recommend that people with diabetes *try* to limit their cholesterol intake to 200 milligrams or less per day because of their increased risk of heart disease.

Remember also that keeping an eye on portion sizes is a key to improved blood glucose.

107

I know it seems rather odd to combine carbohydrates with mono-unsaturated fat, but what I'm really saying is that if you opt for a little less carbohydrate in your diet, make up the difference with monounsaturated (in particular) fat. Remember our sources of monounsaturated fat are primarily olive and canola oils, and avocado. In general, the advice to those with diabetes reiterates the diet recommendations given to all Americans to limit saturated fat and cholesterol-rich foods.

In the pages that follow, you will find tips and tables to help you eat less saturated fat and cholesterol and more monounsaturated fat and to eat more fiber, particularly soluble fiber. You will also find tools to help manage your blood sugar better, such as a comprehensive table listing all of the known glycemic indexes of carbohydrate-containing foods.

BEING YOUR OWN BLOOD GLUCOSE DETECTIVE II: THE DIET DIARY

The best part about being someone with diabetes is that you know what effect a particular meal or snack has on your blood glucose level almost immediately. About an hour and a half after eating, you will know whether your blood sugar is within normal limits, high, or low. This is your greatest tool. Use it.

No matter what master eating strategy you are using to plan your meals, a certain portion of it will always be trial and error because each of us reacts a little differently to food, or a certain combination of foods, and each of us will eat a different amount of those foods. The only way you can learn your own personal reaction to a particular meal is to test your blood sugar an hour and half later.

You cannot become your own blood glucose detective *without* testing your blood sugar regularly. Once you get in the habit of testing your blood sugar after meals, you can look back to your records for clues on why your readings are what they are. As I outlined in the previous chapter, you can look for clues in three possible categories:

1. food and diet (What foods and how much did you eat?)
2. a change in your exercise schedule (Did you exercise at your usual time?)
3. medication (Did you take the proper amount of medication, and was it taken at the proper time?)

So, assuming your exercise hadn't changed that day and your medication was taken correctly, that leaves food and diet. Ask yourself what you ate that was out of the ordinary? Did you eat a larger portion of one particular food?

A Personal Case

My dad told me his blood sugar was really high one afternoon. My first question was "What did you have for lunch?" He told me a few things and then he mentioned that he had watermelon. I asked him, "How much watermelon did you have?" He said about a half. I said, "You mean half of a slice?" and he said, "No, half of a watermelon!"

You see, to say my dad loves watermelon is an understatement. His body probably could have handled a small bowl of watermelon, or even a whole slice of watermelon just fine, but *half a watermelon* was obviously way too much. His blood sugar reminded him that he needed to make sure he ate only a small bowl or slice of watermelon at a time. If he chooses to eat a lot more than that, he can expect very high blood sugar levels about an hour or two later.

Keeping a Diary

As a blood glucose detective, you can use another tool to help piece the puzzle together. You can keep a diary to track:

Your intake: What you ate (and how much), and when you ate it.

Your output: When did you exercise? What did you do and for how long?

Your medication: When did you take any medication? How much did you take?

Your blood levels: What was your blood sugar level at various times during the day?

This daily drudgery can be your biggest ally. At the very least it can help you determine your own personal blood glucose response to various foods or food combinations. You will find a list of the glycemic indexes for all the foods I could find indexes for in the table later in this chapter, but there will still be some individual variation. Keeping track of the food you eat and how your body reacted to it will help you understand what you can do better next time. It can pinpoint your particular trouble spots.

For example, maybe you find your blood sugar tends to get too high after you eat pizza. Next time you eat pizza, try to eat one slice *less* and maybe have some green salad with vegetables and kidney or garbanzo beans instead.

Will this lower your blood sugar response to pizza? Test your blood sugar and you'll have your answer.

THE GLYCEMIC INDEX GUIDE

The glycemic index guide on page 112 is a great tool, but it isn't the "end-all." I wish it was. You will still need to consider the total amount of carbohydrate you eat, the amount and type of fat, and the fiber and salt content of foods. The information in the table is still very helpful.

As I explained in chapter 4, every food is given a number (the glycemic index), or range of numbers, that represents how it affects blood glucose hours after a meal compared to a reference food: either white bread or straight glucose, which is given the number 100. When glucose is used as the reference food (as it is in the table), white bread ends up with a glycemic index of 70. When bread is used as the reference food, glucose has a glycemic index of around 137.

But keep in mind it's never that simple. For instance, you normally eat a particular food in combination with other foods. Well, the presence of fats and proteins has been shown to influence glycemic response to carbohydrates in mixed meals. You also might prepare that food differently from the method indicated in the list. And any process that changes the texture or disrupts the physical or botanical structure of ingredients will change (mostly increase) the plasma glucose and insulin responses.

For example, a recent article reported that all pasta products had signficantly lower glycemic indexes than the reference bread, even though both the pasta and the bread were made from 100 percent durum flour. There seems to be something about the processing and baking of bread that gives it, in general, higher glycemic values than pasta. And while we are on the subject of pasta, some studies found that the more gelatinized or gummy the starch granules, the higher the glycemic index. Is this an endorsement for ordering your pasta "al dente"?

Bread, however, is a another story. With the exception of pumpernickel bread and kernel breads made from wheat, rye, and barley, most bread products, even whole wheat breads, elicit high glucose and insulin responses. When bread is enriched with viscous fiber components such as oat bran or linseed, glucose and insulin responses are reduced. So if bread is enriched with viscous fiber, you may be able to create a bread with a lower glycemic index (and a lower blood sugar response).

The Benefits of "Slow" (or Low Glycemic) Carbohydrates

As I discussed in chapter 4, research has shown that eating primarily low glycemic-index foods can improve overall blood sugar control in people with diabetes. And there's a bonus: some studies have also shown low glycemic index diets reduce serum cholesterol and triglyceride levels. What are called "slow meals"—those made up of lower-glycemic-index carbohydrates—have also been reported to prolong the duration of satiety (or fullness), suggesting a preventive role in obesity. One article reported that as plasma glucose goes up, satiety goes down.

Just remember how satisfied or full you felt shortly after eating a couple of pieces of toast or a bowl of Crispix breakfast cereal. I don't know about you, but in about thirty minutes I have to ask myself, "Did I just eat?"—because my stomach is empty again and I feel like eating. These two breakfasts would not be described as "slow" meals. The glucose response to them will probably be fast and fairly high. A "slower" breakfast might be a bowl of oatmeal with a couple of strips of turkey bacon or a lower-cholesterol vegetable omelette served with an oat bran muffin and a 50 percent less fat Jimmy Dean sausage patty. Those breakfasts are more likely to "stick to your ribs," as the old expression goes, and keep you from midmorning hunger.

What might be most helpful for people with diabetes is that insulin responses to carbohydrate-rich foods tend to follow the rank order of the glycemic responses. That means the foods with the lowest glycemic indexes tend to naturally have the lowest insulin levels following a meal.

Several studies on the glycemic index focused on its usefulness for athletes. Low-glycemic-index foods eaten before prolonged strenuous exercise were found to improve endurance times and resulted in higher concentrations of fuel (energy) in the blood toward the end of exercise.

Whether you are an athlete, someone with diabetes, or simply trying to curb your appetite or lower your blood lipids, the glycemic index of foods may be helpful. As more scientific research is performed, I have a feeling that this information may prove to be even more beneficial. You can use the table to help you detect why you might have high blood sugar after a particular meal. You can also look up the carbohydrate in the meal you just ate to see whether it was high- or low-glycemic. Perhaps all of your carbohydrate foods in that meal had high-glycemic indexes (such as bread and potatoes)? Compare your blood sugar after this meal to a meal when most of your carbohydrate foods had low-glycemic indexes (such as spaghetti noodles and kidney beans).

The Glycemic Index of Foods

(Glucose = 100)

The foods with glycemic indexes of 40 or below are identified with an asterisk (*). These are the items that might be defined as low-glycemic foods.

Beverages

cordial, orange	66	+/– 8	
soft drink, Fanta	68	+/– 6	

Bread

bagel, white (Lender's)	72		
barley flour bread	65		(80 percent barley flour)
bulgur bread	52	+/– 3	
French baguette	95	+/– 15	
mixed-grain bread	45	+/– 7	
oat bran bread	50		(45 percent oat bran)
pita bread	57		
pumpernickel	41		
pumpernickel, whole-grain	46		
rye flour bread	65	+/– 2	
semolina bread	64		
white bread	70		
wheat bread	68	+/– 1	(white, high-fiber)
whole-meal bread	69	+/– 2	

Bun

hamburger bun	61
kaiser rolls	73

Cake

angel food	67	
banana cake	47	+/– 8
pound cake	54	
sponge cake	46	+/– 6

Candy

chocolate	49	+/– 6
jelly beans	80	+/– 8
Life Savers	70	+/– 6
Mars bar	68	+/– 12

Cereals, Cold

All-Bran	42	+/– 5
Bran Buds with Psyllium	47	
Bran Chex	58	
Cheerios	74	
Corn Bran	75	
Corn Chex	83	
Corn Flakes	84	+/– 3
Crispix	87	
Golden Grahams	71	
Grape-Nuts	67	
Grape-Nuts Flakes	80	
Life	66	
Muesli, average	66	+/– 9
Nutri-Grain	66	+/– 12
oat bran, raw	55	+/– 6
puffed wheat	74	+/– 9
rice bran*	19	+/– 3
Rice Chex	89	
Rice Krispies	82	
Shredded Wheat	69	+/– 6
Special K	54	+/– 4
Total	76	

Cereals, Hot

Cream of Wheat	66
Cream of Wheat, Instant	74
Quaker Quick Oats	65

Cookies

graham crackers	74	
oatmeal	54	+/– 4
shortbread	64	+/– 8
tea cookies	55	+/– 4
vanilla wafers	77	

Crackers

Kavli Norwegian Crispbread	71	+/– 7
melba toast (Old London)	70	
rice cakes	82	+/– 11

(continued)

Stoned Wheat Thins	67		
water crackers	72	+/– 4	
croissant	67		

Desserts, Other

custard	43	+/– 10	milk + starch + sugar
doughnut, cake-type	76		

Fruit

apple*	36	+/– 2
apricots, canned, in light syrup	64	
apricots, dried*	31	+/– 1
banana	53	+/– 6
cherries*	22	
cocktail, fruit, canned	55	
grapefruit*	25	
grapes	43	
kiwi fruit	52	+/– 6
mango	55	+/– 5
orange	43	+/– 4
peach, fresh*	28	
peach, canned, in light syrup	52	
pear*	36	+/– 3
pears, canned, in pear juice	44	
pineapple	66	+/– 7
plum*	24	
raisins	64	+/– 11
sultanas	56	+/– 11
watermelon	72	+/– 13

Fruit Juice

apple juice	41	+/– 1	unsweetened
grapefruit juice	48		unsweetened
orange juice	57	+/– 3	
pineapple juice	46		unsweetened

Grains

barley*, regular and pearled	25	+/– 2
barley, cracked	50	
barley, rolled	66	+/– 5
buckwheat	54	+/– 4

bulgur, boiled 20 minutes	48	+/– 2	
couscous	65	+/– 6	
cornmeal	68		
millet	71	+/– 10	
rice, white, long-grain	56	+/– 2	boiled
rice, white, low-amylose	88	+/– 3	(Waxy, Calrose, Pelde rice growers)
rice, white, high-amylose	59	+/– 3	(Basmati, Doongara rice growers)
rice, brown	55	+/– 5	
rice, parboiled, average	47	+/– 3	(i.e., Uncle Ben's Converted)
rice, wild (Saskatchewan)	57		
rice, Mexican	58		(Uncle Ben's Fast and Fancy)
rye*, whole kernel	34	+/– 3	
tapioca boiled with milk	81		
wheat, whole kernel	41	+/– 3	

Ice Cream

average	61	+/– 7
ice cream, low-fat	50	+/– 8

Legumes

baked beans, canned	48	+/– 8
black-eyed peas	42	+/– 9
butter beans*	31	+/– 3
chick-peas (garbanzo beans)*	33	+/– 1
chick-peas, canned	42	
haricot (navy) beans*	38	+/– 6
kidney beans*	27	+/– 5
kidney beans, canned	52	
lentils, green*	30	+/– 4
lentils, green, canned	52	
lentils, red*	26	+/– 4
lima beans, baby, frozen*	32	
pinto beans*	39	
pinto beans, canned	45	
Romano beans	46	
soy beans*	18	+/– 3

(continued)

| soy beans, canned* | 14 | +/– 2 |
| split peas, yellow, boiled* | 32 | |

Milk

milk, whole*	27	+/– 7
milk, skim*	32	+/– 5
milk, chocolate, sweetened*	34	+/– 4
milk, chocolate, artificially sweetened*	24	+/– 6

Muffins

apple muffin	44	+/– 6	
bran muffin	60		
blueberry muffin	59		
carrot muffin	62		
corn muffin	49		(high-amylose cornmeal used)

Nuts

| peanuts* | 14 | +/– 8 |

Pasta

capellini	45		
fettuccine, egg-enriched*	32	+/– 4	
instant noodles	47		
linguine, thick	46	+/– 3	made with durum wheat
linguine, thin	55	+/– 6	made with durum wheat
macaroni, boiled 5 minutes	45		
macaroni and cheese	64		Kraft from box
ravioli, meat-filled*	39	+/– 1	made with durum wheat
rice vermicelli	58		
spaghetti	41	+/– 3	boiled an average of 15 minutes
spaghetti, boiled 5 minutes*	37	+/– 3	
spaghetti, whole-meal*	37	+/– 5	
spirali, made with durum	43	+/– 10	
star pastina, boiled 5 minutes*	38		
tortellini, cheese-filled	50		Stouffer
vermicelli*	35	+/– 7	

Pastry	**59**	**+/– 6**	
Sausage*	**28**	**+/– 6**	
Snack Foods			
corn chips	73	+/– 1	
popcorn	55	+/– 7	
potato crisps	54	+/– 3	
Soups			
black bean	64		
green pea, canned	66		Campbell Soup
lentil, canned	44		Unico, Culinar Foods Inc.
split pea	60		Wil-Pak Foods
tomato*	38	+/– 9	
Sugars			
honey	73	+/– 15	
fructose*	23	+/– 1	
glucose	97	+/– 3	
glucose tablets, Glucodin	102	+/– 9	
maltose	105	+/– 12	
sucrose	65	+/– 4	
lactose	46	+/– 3	
Stuffing, Bread	**74**		
Taco Shells	**68**		
Tofu			
Vegetables			
carrots	71	+/– 22	
corn, sweet	55	+/– 1	
green peas	48	+/– 5	
parsnips	97	+/– 19	
potato, instant	83	+/– 1	

(continued)

potato, baked	85	+/– 12	made without fat
potato, French fries	75		Cavendish Farms, Prince Edward Island
potato, new	62	+/– 7	
potato, mashed	70	+/– 2	
potato, boiled	56	+/– 1	
pumpkin	75	+/– 9	
rutabaga	72	+/– 8	
sweet potato	54	+/– 8	
yam	51	+/– 12	

Waffles, Aunt Jemima	**76**	

Yogurt

yogurt, low-fat, fruit*	33	+/– 7	sugar sweetened
yogurt, low-fat*	14	+/– 4	artificial sweetener

Indigenous Foods

Pima Indian Foods

acorns, stewed with venison*	16	+/– 1
cactus jam	91	
corn hominy*	40	+/– 5
fruit leather	70	
lima bean broth*	36	+/– 3
mesquite cakes*	25	+/– 3
tortilla*	38	

Mexican Foods

black beans*	30
brown beans*	38
nopal, prickly pear cactus*	7

Asian-Indian Foods

baisen chapati*	27		
bajra	57	+/– 5	
banana, unripe	70	+/– 11	steamed 1 hour
barley chapati	42	+/– 5	
bengal gram dhal, chick-pea*	11		
black gram	43	+/– 10	
green gram*	38	+/– 14	

Source: © 1995 *The American Journal of Clinical Nutrition* 62: 871S–93S, American Society for Clinical Nutrition. Used with permission.

TIMING YOUR MEDICATION AND MEALS

Eating proper portion sizes helps keep calorie levels consistent. And when calories are consistent and mealtimes are consistent, blood glucose control is usually not far away. Work with your dietitian or certified diabetes educator to make sure, when your meal plan is being designed, that your meals are scheduled at a practical time for you. Eating meals at nearly the same time each day will help in your blood glucose management, especially if you are also taking medication or insulin for your diabetes.

HOW TO STOP BAD SNACKING HABITS

Having a healthy relationship with food is a wonderful goal. To me, this means eating when you are hungry and stopping when you are comfortably full. It sounds simple. It started out simple when we were newborns. But for many of us it isn't simple anymore. Years of dieting have taught many of us to do exactly the opposite—*not* to eat when we are hungry, which led to feelings of deprivation and intense hunger. We started ignoring our natural hunger and satiety signals, which led to *not* stopping when we were comfortably full.

As an entire nation, we need to get off the dieting train and get back to the basics of eating when we are hungry and stopping when we are comfortably full. But for many of us some damage has already been done. We tend either to overeat certain foods or we overeat during certain situations.

Are there foods that you tend to overeat? When you are in the presence of these foods, you can't seem to stop? What if you let yourself have some every time you were truly hungry and had a hankering for it? Would that stop you from going overboard as before? This strategy might work for some people.

I met a woman who said every time she came near a box of Sees chocolates she would fast and furiously end up eating the whole box. I asked her if this was something she often wanted but deprived herself of. She said yes. I suggested she lift the ban and work a piece or two into her normal eating shedule on the days when she wanted it. Months later she told me it had been working out great. She doesn't seem to want them as often and she hasn't overeaten them since. This situation reminds me of the saying "absence makes the heart grow fonder." When you deprive yourself of something you want, it only makes you want it more.

For other people or other foods, the saying "out of sight, out of mind" might be more appropriate. It certainly applies to my dad, who ends up eating half the watermelon each time he buys one. He finds it best to simply not buy them. He enjoys a more reasonable portion of watermelon when it is served to him at a restaurant or at my house. I asked him if this makes him feel deprived. He said, "No, as long as I can still have it sometimes."

Are there certain situations or cues that encourage you to eat when you really aren't hungry or eat past the point of comfortable fullness? Here's one example when most of us do. We have just enjoyed a wonderful meal. We are comfortably full, perhaps sipping a cup of tea or coffee. Out comes the dessert. It is so appealing you can't refuse a piece even though you aren't hungry anymore. The way I see it, you have three options here. One, you can stuff a big piece down anyway. Two, you can ask to take a piece home (if you are at someone else's house or a restaurant) or save a piece for later (if you are at your own home). Or, three, you can ask for a sampler-size piece, just to enjoy a bite or two of the dessert with your coffee.

I tend to do the last. After all, I'm interested in the dessert now, but I'm not hungry. So what I really want is "tasting," not "eating," the dessert. If it's so wonderful I want more than a taste, I put a piece away for later, when I am hungry. I admit, though, being satisfied with a "taste" and putting a piece aside for later is easier for some people than others. The truth is we enjoy our food better when we are truly hungry. Do you remember how great food tastes when you are camping? When we are camping, we are more active than usual: walking, hiking and swimming, breathing in fresh air, and becoming noticeably hungry before each meal, particularly breakfast.

Some of us tend to overeat during emotionally stressful times when we are feeling angry, lonely, or depressed. Food offers only temporary relief from the pain. Stress-related bingeing is more likely to be a snack time (not a mealtime) behavior. It is more likely to be done in private and is more often done by women than by men. Some studies have reported the incidence of emotional eating in overweight people to be as high as three out of four individuals.

If you think you are an emotional eater, you might need to work through some of your stresses and emotions with a counselor. In general, to help emotional eating go away, you need to work through the emotional stressors so they occur less often and are less significant when they do, and find more healthful and productive ways of coping with these stressors when they arise. Entire books are written on this subject, so obviously I can't sufficiently cover the issue here. Try to get the help you need. You might start by talking with a sympathetic member of your health care team.

Discouraging overeating episodes will improve your diabetes in the short and long term. When you relearn to eat when you are hungry and stop when you are comfortably full, your blood glucose will be easier to manage day by day. And when you avoid overeating, you're more likely to achieve that moderate weight loss (if you are presently overweight), improving your diabetes management and reducing your health risks for the future.

FREE FOODS FOR ANY TIME OF DAY (OR NIGHT)

You've got the nibbles. You feel like gnawing on something, but it isn't time for you to eat a meal or snack. Perhaps it is the middle of the night. Maybe it's an hour before dinner. What do you do? Find a "free" food, or "almost free" food, to eat or drink. Of course, I don't mean free in the sense that it doesn't cost money. Food is virtually "free" to a person with diabetes when it contributes very few calories and carbo grams. It doesn't need to be counted; it can be eaten any time of day or night.

I'll be honest with you. There isn't an abundance of "free" foods to choose from. You have your predictable sugar-free Jell-O or sugar-free candies you can suck on (two of the sugar-free type of hard candy contribute around 50 calories and 12 grams of carbohydrate). You have raw vegetables to crunch and fat-free dips to make them a little more exciting. You can freeze sugar-free lemonade to make lemonade ice or lemonade pops, which are not only "free" but particularly refreshing during hot summer months (each cup of lemonade ice might contribute 1 to 2 grams of carbohydrate).

I am not a sugar-free Jell-O fan, but I tried to work up a few "almost free" recipes to make it appetizing—even to me. You'll find these recipes below. And the fat-free dips listed below are easy to make and tasty too.

A few "almost free" products and recipes are also worth mentioning, if only to give you a few more options in the middle of the night when the mood hits. Let's face it, there may be times when sugar-free Jell-O or raw vegetables just don't cut it. Perhaps sugar-free chocolate pudding sounds more like it (made with skim or lowfat milk). A half cup serving will cost you 80 calories (made with skim or low-fat milk) and 15 grams of carbohydrate. It's not "free," but it's better than a couple of slices of bread, which will pump 140 calories and 24 grams of carbohydrate into your bloodstream.

Sugar-free Fudgsicles (Good Humor) can be kept in the freezer for just such occasions when you have a hankering for a treat or snack at the wrong time of day. One of these will run you about 40 calories and 8 grams of carbohydrate. A cup of sugar-free hot cocoa usually contains 40 calories and less than 10 grams of carbohydrate.

FREE AND ALMOST-FREE RECIPES

Lemonade Ice

2 cups sugar-free lemonade

Pour lemonade into an ice cube tray, leaving room at the top for the lemonade to expand while freezing. Place tray in freezer. The lemonade ice will be ready to eat in about an hour. Place a cup of the lemonade ice cubes in an ice crusher, ice shaver, or blender, and grind, shave, or chop until ice flakes form. Serve in cups with a spoon. You can pop out the ice cubes and store them in a Ziploc bag in the freezer until you need them.

This snack contributes about 1 to 2 grams of carbohydrate per 1-cup serving.

Chocolate Pudding

Makes 6 servings

3 cups cold skim or low-fat milk
1 package chocolate Jell-O sugar-free Instant Pudding (2.1 ounces)

Pour milk into a medium bowl. Add mix. Beat with electric mixer on lowest speed for 2 minutes. Pour at once into 6 dessert dishes. Refrigerate until ready to serve (it should be soft set in 5 minutes).

Per serving: 80 calories, 15 g carbohydrate, 0 g fat, 1 g fiber, 384 mg sodium, 0 mg cholesterol

Note: Sugar-free pudding also comes in butterscotch, vanilla, and banana cream.

Lemon Whip

Makes 4 servings

1 package sugar-free lemon Jell-O (.3 ounce)
1 cup boiling water
Ice cubes
6 ounces low-fat or light (with NutraSweet) lemon yogurt
1/2 cup Light Cool Whip, Dream Whip, or pressurized light whipped cream (optional)

In a 4-cup measure, stir Jell-O powder with boiling water for 2 minutes, or until completely dissolved. Add ice cubes to mixture until it measures 2 cups. Stir until ice cubes dissolve. Stir or beat in lemon yogurt. Spoon into 4 dessert dishes, and refrigerate 4 hours, or until firm. Decorate each serving with a dollop (2 tablespoons) of Light Cool Whip, Dream Whip, or light whipped cream, if desired.

Per serving:
- *With low-fat yogurt:* 55 calories, 2.7 g protein, 8 g carbohydrate, .4 g fat, .2 g saturated fat, 86 mg sodium, 2 mg cholesterol
- *With light yogurt (and NutraSweet):* 10 calories, 1 g protein, 0 g carbohydrate, 0 g fat, 0 g saturated fat, 55 mg sodium, 0 mg cholesterol
- *With topping (added to above totals):* 20 calories, 2 g fat, 1 g saturated fat, 5 mg cholesterol

Low-Fat Ranch Dip

My favorite light sour cream is Naturally Yours, the one in the cowhide container. Best Foods/Hellmann's makes a good light mayonnaise, which can be used instead of regular mayonnaise in this recipe. I find that regular mayonnaise helps balance the flavors in this recipe.

Makes 1 cup
1/2 packet Hidden Valley Original Ranch Party Dip
1 cup fat-free sour cream
1 tablespoon mayonnaise

> Raw vegetables: carrots, celery, jicama, zucchini, and so on. Stir contents of the half packet gently into sour cream and mayonnaise. Mix with a wire whisk or a spoon. Refrigerate for 1 hour before serving, if possible. Serve with your favorite raw vegetables.
>
> **Per serving:** 2 tablespoons dip with 1/2 carrot and 1/2 large celery stalk, cut into sticks—67 calories, 10 g carbohydrate, 1.5 g fat, 1.5 g fiber, 272 mg sodium, 1 mg cholesterol

Low-Fat French Onion Dip

Makes about 1 cup
1/2 envelope Lipton Recipe Secrets Onion Soup Mix (or similar)
1 cup fat-free sour cream
1 tablespoon BestFoods/Hellman's mayonnaise
Raw vegetables: carrot, celery, jicama, zucchini, and so on.

In small bowl, blend all ingredients; chill at least 1 hour. Serve with your favorite raw vegetables.

> **Per serving:** 2 tablespoons dip and 1 stalk celery, cut into sticks—65 calories, 10 g carbohydrate, 1.5 g fat, 1.5 g fiber, 138 mg sodium, 1 mg cholesterol

MORE ON MONOUNSATURATED AND SATURATED FAT

Monounsaturated fat is "in" for the moment, and saturated fat is still "out." This shift is the result of dietary research rather than culinary fashion. So, for good reasons, if you have to choose a fat for a recipe, monounsaturated fat is best. While recent discoveries have been leading us down a Mediterranean path (see below), research has also been supporting the idea of keeping saturated fat at a comfortable minimum. This is a tough one for Americans.

The biggest contributor of saturated fat and cholesterol in the American diet is the meat group, which includes beef, processed meats, eggs, poultry, and other meats. In general, if you choose lower-fat or leaner meats and fat-free egg substitutes and take the skin off the poultry, you will also be lowering the amount of saturated fat and cholesterol.The second largest saturated fat contributor is the milk group. When you choose reduced-fat or low-fat dairy options, you also reduce your intake of saturated fat and cholesterol.

When it comes to eating less saturated fat and cholesterol, you've heard it all before. But what's all this hoopla about possibly eating more monounsaturated fat? For examples of how to eat more monounsaturated fat while eating less saturated fat and cholesterol, look across the ocean to the Mediterranean countries and their cuisine.

AMERICANIZING THE MEDITERRANEAN DIET

By now, most of us have heard about the heart disease prevention benefits of the Mediterranean diet. We may have read about how health organizations are encouraging the general population to mimic Mediterranean meals more often, with their right kind of fat and ample fruits and vegetables. But most of us really don't have any idea what kinds of foods and dishes are actually eaten along the Mediterranean sea, aside from a heavy reliance on olive oil.

The heavy use of olive oil may be of particular interest to people with diabetes, since the new ADA diabetes nutrition guidelines suggest limiting saturated fat and cholesterol while increasing monounsaturated fats as needed to find the right balance of fat and carbohydrate for each particular person. Enter olive oil.

The Mediterranean diet keeps servings of red meat small and infrequent, compared to a heavy use of fish and shellfish, beans, and vegetables, which contribute protein without quite as much saturated fat and cholesterol. The main Mediterranean crops are wheat, olives, and grapes, and these ingredients strongly define the dishes of the various regions. In general, Mediterranean dishes go heavy on the cereals and grains, fruits and vegetables, and fish while limiting dairy products and meats, although poultry is popular.

If you go to the bookstore in search of a Mediterranean cookbook in the hopes of it helping you "Mediterraneanize" your American diet, you will have few choices. But some of these recipes require the kind of time, ingredients, and food tastes that most Americans just don't have. So, using a classic Mediterranean cookbook for inspiration, I Americanized a few recipes I thought might be most likely to go over with Americans. You'll find these recipes in chapter 8.

The following are the main nutritional attributes of the Mediterranean way of eating.

Switch to Mostly Monounsaturated Fats

Where Americans use butter, Mediterraneans use olive oil. Yes, even on bread. When buying olive oil, choose a pungent, deep green, extra-virgin, cold-pressed olive oil for better quality and flavor.

Avocados

Avocados are rich in monounsaturated fats. Eating avocados is not a problem for me—I love them. Just make sure you apportion no more than one-quarter of a whole avocado for each person. Even though some might consider this serving size of avocado small, it already contains 81 calories and 7.7 grams of fat (albeit mostly monounsaturated).

Go Fishing

For many Americans, the only fish they eat is the occasional tuna salad or a fish sandwich from a fast-food restaurant. In the Mediterranean, fish is often served with pasta, rice, or even bread. Shellfish is also commonly featured in recipes, including crab, squid, shrimp, mussels, lobster, oyster, clams, and scallops. You will also find recipes for fish such as sea bass, anchovies, swordfish, monkfish, tuna, and mullet. Sardines and mackerel are particularly popular, and are served either baked or broiled. You will find a few quick and delicious recipes for fish and shellfish in chapter 8.

Eat Your Fruits and Vegetables

Even kids in the Mediterranean rarely have to be reminded to eat their vegetables, because vegetables are such a big part of Mediterranean cuisine. Mediterranean recipes include vegetables such as fresh and dried mushrooms, broccoli, cauliflower, cabbage, leeks, onions, carrots, turnips, spinach and salad greens, winter squash and pumpkins, celery, asparagus, peppers, artichokes, eggplant, tomatoes, cucumbers, zucchini, and fennel. Many of these vegetables are also available (some of them year round) in the United States.

Fruits such as strawberries, peaches, pears, lemons, oranges, watermelon and other melons, apples, grapes, plums, pomegranates, fresh figs, and dried fruit are common in the Meditteranean, as are pine nuts, almonds, walnuts, hazelnuts, chestnuts, and olives.

Besides olive oil, there is one flavor you will find consistently throughout Mediterranean cooking—garlic. As I thumbed through Mediterranean cookbooks, I rarely met a main course recipe that didn't have it—and a lot of it. Garlic is not only a great way to add flavor without adding fat and calories, it may just be a health-promoting substance in its own right because of the plant chemicals it naturally contains (phytochemicals), which may discourage the growth of cancerous tumors. Large amounts of garlic may also contribute to lowering lipids.

Better Buy Beans

Americans go so far as to have beans in their chili and beans with their Mexican food, but that's about the extent of our bean cuisine. Mediterraneans add beans to soup, pasta, and rice dishes as well as various entrees. Barlotti beans and fava beans, chick-peas, lentils, and white beans are the beans you'll find most in Mediterranean recipes. Not only do beans and peas contribute protein, they are low in fat, and, probably most important, they are bursting with soluble fiber and phytochemicals.

Do you want to know how to boost your soluble fiber quickly and painlessly, short of making an oat bran shake or eating several oat bran muffins? Better buy beans. A half cup of beans will offer from 6 to11 grams of fiber, mostly soluble fiber. You'll find a few delicious bean recipes in chapter 8.

Other Tidbits (Use If You Like, Where You Can)

Mediterraneans make some grain dishes that we're not used to here in America, such as bulghur wheat, semolina, and couscous. But we are, at least, quite familiar with the culinary delights of rice and pasta, which are staples in the Mediterranean.

Wine (sherry, marsala) and vinegar (wine, sherry, and balsamic vinegars) are commonly used in Mediterranean recipes. Sheep and goat's milk are often used to make cheese. The following are the cheeses you are probably most likely to recognize: feta, ricotta, mozzarella (though in the Mediterranean it is made from buffalo milk), pecorino (similar to Parmesan but made from sheep's milk), Parmesan, and gorgonzola.

Some other ingredients that help define Mediterranean cuisine are tahini (made from crushed sesame seeds), red hot chili paste, honey, anchovies, green and black olives, pimiento, and sun-dried tomatoes.

MAKING FIBER YOUR FRIEND

One of the keys to a high-carbohydrate eating plan for someone with diabetes is that meals are also high in fiber, particularly soluble fiber. We've talked about 30 to 40 grams of fiber as a goal. But just how easy it that, really?

The Quickest Way to 30 or 40 Grams of Fiber

- A serving of beans every day, at lunch or dinner
- A high-fiber cereal every day, at breakfast or as a snack
- A high-oat-bran food (or oatmeal) every day
- At least 5 servings of high-fiber fruits and vegetables every day
- *Perhaps for some,* a serving of a high-fiber supplement (consult your doctor or dietitian first)

Could you do it? For a list of the higher-fiber foods, see the following table. A little help with the fiber math, which might make the task a little less daunting, follows.

Higher-Fiber Foods

The following foods have 4 grams or more fiber per practical serving. In order to make it easier to count carbohydrate and fat while trying to emphasize these higher-fiber foods, grams of fat and carbohydrate have been included in this table.

	Fiber (g)	Carbo-hydrate (g)	Fat (g)	Calories
Fruits				
apple with peel, large (7.5 oz.)	4.0	32.0	0.8	125
blackberries/boysenberries, 1 cup	6.5	18.0	0.5	75
orange, sections, 1 1/4 cup	4.3	26.0	0.3	106
pear, D'Anjou, large (7.4 oz.)	5.0	32.0	0.8	123
raspberries, 1 cup	5.0	14.0	0.7	60
Vegetables				
artichoke globe, boiled	6.5	13.0	0.2	60
artichoke hearts, 1/2 cup, water-packed	5.0	9.0	0.1	37
asparagus pieces, 1 cup cooked	4.0	7.5	0.5	43
broccoli pieces, 1 cup boiled	5.0	8.0	0.5	44
Brussels sprouts, 1 cup cooked	7.0	13.5	0.8	61
carrots, 1 cup cooked	4.0	16.5	0.3	70
green beans, 1 cup boiled	4.0	10.0	0.3	44
green peas, 1/2 cup cooked	4.5	12.5	0.2	67
greens, turnip, frozen,1 cup cooked	4.5	6.5	0.3	29
greens, chicory, 1 cup raw	7.0	8.5	0.5	41
greens, dock/sorrel, 1 cup raw, chopped	4.0	4.5	1.0	29
parsnips, 1 cup boiled	7.0	30.5	0.5	126
potato, 1 large with skin	5.0	51.0	0.2	220
snow peas, frozen, 1 cup cooked	3.0	6.0	0.1	20
spinach, frozen, 1 cup cooked	5.0	10.0	0.4	53
spinach, 2 1/2 cups chopped fresh	4.0	5.0	0.5	31
squash, acorn, 1/2 cup cooked cubes	4.5	15.0	0.1	58
succotash, 1/2 cup boiled	5.0	23.5	0.8	110
yams, 1 cup cooked cubes	5.0	37.5	0.2	158

	Fiber (g)	Carbo- hydrate (g)	Fat (g)	Calories
Beans and Bean Products				
baby lima beans, 1/2 cup cooked	4.5	20.0	0.3	105
black beans, 1/2 cup canned	7.0	17.0	1.0	100
black-eyed peas, 1/2 cup boiled	4.0	17.0	0.3	80
Great Northern beans, 1/2 cup cooked	5.0	18.5	0.4	104
kidney beans, 1/2 cup canned	8.0	20.0	0.4	109
lima beans, 1/2 cup canned	4.0	15.5	0.3	82
navy beans, 1/2 cup cooked	8.0	24.0	0.5	129
pinto beans, 1/2 cup canned	7.0	18.0	1.0	110
pork and beans, 1/2 cup canned in tomato sauce	6.0	24.5	1.5	124
pork and beans, 1/2 cup canned in sweet sauce	5.5	26.5	2.0	140
refried beans, 1/2 cup canned	7.0	23.5	1.5	136
white beans, 1/2 cup canned	6.5	28.5	0.4	153
Canned Bean Products				
Bush's Vegetarian Baked Beans, 1/2 cup (550 mg sodium)	6.0	24.0	0	130
Campbell's Pork & Beans, 1/2 cup (420 mg sodium)	6.0	24.0	2.0	130
chili with beans, 1/2 cup canned	5.5	15.0	7.0	143
Dennison's Vegetarian Chili, 1 cup (1,080 mg sodium)	9.0	35.0	1.0	180
Heinz Vegetarian Beans, 1/2 cup (480 mg sodium)	5.0	27.0	0.5	140
Hormel Vegetarian Chili, 1 cup (830 mg sodium)	9.0	38.0	0	200
Rosarita No Fat Traditional Refried beans, 1/2 cup (550 mg sodium)	5.0	19.0	0	100
Rosarita Zest No Fat Refried beans, 1/2 cup (550 mg sodium)	8.0	22.0	0	100
Townhouse Vegetarian Refried beans, 1/2 cup (440 mg sodium)	8.0	23.0	1.0	135

(continued)

	Fiber (g)	Carbo-hydrate (g)	Fat (g)	Calories
Bread products				
pumpernickel bread, 2 slices	4.5	30.5	2.0	160
whole wheat bread, 2 slices	4.5	32.0	3.0	172
oat bran bread, 2 slices	5.0	23.5	2.5	140
Orowheat Light country oat bread (with oats and oat fiber), 2 slices	5.0	18	0.5	80
Cold Cereals				
All-Bran, $1/2$ cup	10.0	22.0	1.0	80
All-Bran Extra Fiber, $1/2$ cup	15.0	22.0	1.0	50
Almond Delight, 1 cup	4.0	41.0	3.0	210
Banana Nut Crunch, 1 cup	4.0	43.0	6.0	250
Blueberry Muesli, 1 cup	4.0	41.0	2.5	200
Bran Buds, $1/2$ cup	16.0	32.5	1.0	111
Chex, Multi Bran, $1 1/4$ cup	7.0	48.0	1.0	220
Chex, Whole Grain, $3/4$ cup	5.0	41.0	1.0	190
Complete Bran Flakes, $3/4$ cup	5.0	24.0	0.5	90
Cracklin' Oat Bran, $3/4$ cup	6.0	40.0	8.0	230
Crispy Wheat 'n Raisins, 1 cup	4.0	44.0	1.0	190
Crunchy Corn Bran, $3/4$ cup	5.0	23.0	1.0	90
Fiber One, $1/2$ cup	13.0	24.0	1.0	60
Frosted Mini-Wheats, 1 cup	5.0	41.0	1.0	170
Frosted Mini-Wheats, 1 cup bite-size	6.0	48.0	1.0	200
Fruit & Fibre, Dates and Walnuts, 1 cup	5.0	40.0	3.0	200
Fruitful Bran, 1 cup	7.0	43.5	0	170
Granola, Kellogg's Low-Fat with raisins, 1 cup	4.5	64.0	4.5	315
Granola, Kellogg's Low-Fat without raisins, 1 cup	6.0	88.0	6.0	420
Granola, Nature Valley Low Fat Fruit Granola, 1 cup	4.5	65.0	4.0	315
Grape-Nuts, $1/2$ cup	5.0	45.0	0.2	194
Grape-Nuts Flakes, whole wheat and barley, $3/4$ cup	4.0	32.0	1.5	133
Healthy Choice Toasted Brown Sugar Squares, 1 cup	5.0	44.0	1.0	190
Kellogg's Bran Flakes, $3/4$ cup	5.0	24.0	0.5	100
Post Bran Flakes, 1 cup	9.0	37.0	1.0	152
Mueslix Raisin and Almond Crunch, $2/3$ cup	4.0	42.0	3.0	200

	Fiber (g)	Carbo-hydrate (g)	Fat (g)	Calories
Nutri-Grain Almond Raisin, 1¼ cup	4.0	38.0	3.0	180
Nutri-Grain Golden Wheat, ¾ cup	4.0	24.0	1.0	100
Oatmeal Squares, Quaker, 1 cup	4.0	43.0	2.5	220
100% Bran, ⅓ cup	8.0	23.0	0.5	80
Quaker 100% Natural Low Fat, 1 cup	4.5	66.0	4.5	315
Raisin Bran, Kellogg's, 1 cup	8.0	47.0	1.5	200
Raisin Bran, Post, 1 cup	8.0	47.0	1.0	190
Raisin Nut Bran, 1 cup	5.0	41.0	4.5	210
Raisin Squares, ¾ cup	5.0	44.0	1.0	180
Shredded Wheat, 2 biscuits	5.0	37.5	0.6	166
Shredded Wheat 'n Bran, 1¼ cups	8.0	47.0	1.0	200
Shredded Wheat Spoonsize, 1 cup	5.0	41.0	0.5	170
Toasted Oatmeal, Quaker, 1¼ cup	4.0	44.0	2.0	210
Total Raisin Bran, 1 cup	5.0	43.0	1.0	180
Total, Whole Grain, 1 cup	4.0	32.0	1.5	146

Hot Cereal

corn grits, 1 cup	4.5	31.5	0.5	145
oatmeal, 1 cup homemade	4.0	25.5	2.5	145
oatmeal, instant, 1½ cups	6.0	36.0	3.5	208
oatmeal, instant, 2 packets maple and brown sugar	6.0	60.0	3.0	300

Grain Products

barley, ½ cup cooked	7.0	30.0	1.0	135
barley, pearl, ½ cup cooked	4.0	22.0	0.5	97
bulgur wheat, ½ cup cooked	4.0	17.0	0.2	76
crackers, Wasa Crisp rye, 6	4.5	39.0	0.6	176
oat bran, ⅓ cup	5.0	20.5	2.0	76
Krusteaz Lite Oat Bran Pancake Mix, three 4-inch pancakes (390 mg sodium)	7.0	35.0	1.0	140
pancakes, whole wheat, 3	5.0	46.0	10.0	324
wheat bran, ¼ cup	6.5	10.0	0.6	32

Canned Soups (per 1 cup)

Campbell's

Chunky Bean 'n' Ham (880 mg sodium)	9.0	29.0	2.0	190

(continued)

	Fiber (g)	Carbo-hydrate (g)	Fat (g)	Calories
Split Pea with Ham and Bacon (860 mg sodium)	5.0	28.0	3.5	180
Campbell's Home Cookin Fiesta Soup (750 mg sodium)	4.0	24.0	2.5	130
Salsa Bean (730 mg sodium)	7.0	31.0	1.0	160
Savory Lentil (860 mg sodium)	5.0	24.0	0.5	130
Tuscany-Style Minestrone	5.0	21.0	7.0	160
Progresso				
Beef Barley (780 mg sodium)	3.0	13.0	4.0	130
Hearty Black Bean (730 mg sodium)	10	30.0	1.5	170
Lentil (750 mg sodium)	7.0	22.0	2.0	140
White Meat Chicken Barley (720 mg sodium)	3.0	13.0	2.0	100
Mixed Dishes				
bean burrito	4.0	36.0	6.5	224
beef and bean burrito grande	5.0	53.0	16	430
moussaka (lamb and eggplant), 1 cup	4.0	14.0	9.0	209
pizza, thick-crust, 1/2 of 10-inch pie	4.0	75.0	10	484
tostada with beans	7.0	26.0	10	223
toastada with beans and chicken or beef	4.0	19.0	11.5	253

DO THE MATH

Some scientists say that 30 to 40 grams of fiber, a large portion of which is soluble fiber, is too impractical for most Americans. There's only one way to find out—let's do the math ourselves.

What if:

- You had some oats *every day*? For example, what if you had a cup of oatmeal, or a cup of a cold oat cereal (oat squares or low-fat granola, etc.), or a couple of slices of oat bran bread, or a serving of oat bran pancakes? You would add *4 to 6 grams of fiber.*
- You ate a few fruits and vegetables *every day*? For example, what if you ate an apple, a carrot, and a cup of cooked green vegetable (like broccoli)? You would add about 4, 4, and 5 grams of fiber, respectively, or *13 grams of fiber* total.

- You ate a serving of beans *every day*? For example, what if you had $^1/_2$ cup of pinto or kidney beans in a salad, or in Mexican food, or in a casserole or soup or chili? You would add about *8 grams of fiber.*

If you just did those three things every day—eat an oat bran–type food, eat a few fruits and vegetables, and eat some beans—you would be at about 27 grams of fiber. Throw in half a cup of All-Bran, Fiber One, or Bran Buds cereal, and you are at or have passed 40 grams of fiber. Can it be done? Definitely. Is it easy? It can be, especially if you like oats, beans, and produce.

What if you don't have a lot of time? Opening a bag of oat bran bread, or a package of instant oatmeal, or a box of oat cereal doesn't take much time at all. Opening a can of beans to add to some soup or salad, or ordering beans at Taco Bell or a Mexican restaurant, doesn't have to be time consuming. Pulling an apple and a carrot from the refrigerator and microwaving a cup of broccoli doesn't have to take too much time either. For more timely tips to pump up your fiber total, as well as keep carbohydrates in balance, see the mealtime tips below.

MEALTIME TIPS—BREAKFAST

The morning is one of the toughest times to keep your blood sugar within normal range. So what and how much you eat for breakfast become particularly important. You need to stick closely to the amount of carbohydrate grams your health care team has outlined in your eating plan. And you will need to avoid a breakfast composed almost entirely of carbohydrate, like a bagel and juice or toast and jam. Better to balance those carbohydrates with some protein and fat. And keeping your breakfast fairly high in soluble fiber may help you as well.

If you really like having pancakes for breakfast, I would try a box of the Lite Oat Bran pancake mix, or some of the oat bran breakfast recipes in chapter 8. Pair those oat bran pancakes with some reduced-fat sausage or turkey bacon and you've got yourself breakfast. Oat bran muffins can be kept in the freezer for a quick-fix breakfast. Just microwave for a minute or two.

If you are going to have toast or a bagel for breakfast, definitely spread it with something contributing protein and fat (to help balance the carbohydrate from the bagel). Peanut butter, light cream cheese, or reduced fat cheese and a couple of slices of ham will do just fine.

See what a difference adding a soluble fiber or adding a protein and fat-rich food will make. Some before and after nutritional profiles are provided below.

Comparing Profiles

Before	After
Plain bagel, 3.5 inch diameter (2.4 oz.)	**Bagel with 1 oz. each of cheese and ham**
36 g carbohydrate (79% of calories)	37 g carbohydrate (49% of calories)
7 g protein (16% of calories)	21 g protein (28% of calories)
1 g fat (5% of calories)	7.5 g fat (23% of calories)
2 slices cracked wheat toast	**2 slices Orowheat Light Country Oat Bread and scrambled eggs (made with Egg Beaters egg substitute, no-stick cooking spray, black pepper, and some herbs)**
31.5 g carbohydrates (79% of calories)	27.5 g carbohydrate (47% of calories)
4 g protein (11% of calories)	20 g protein (34% of calories)
2 g fat (10% of calories)	6.5 g fat (25% of calories)
3.3 g fiber	6 g fiber
3 pancakes plus 1 Tb. syrup	**3 oat bran pancakes with less-fat turkey sausage (3 oz. raw) plus 1 Tb. syrup**
45 g carbohydrates (84% of calories)	45 g carbohydrates (50% of calories)
4 g protein (8% of calories)	20 g protein (23% of calories)
2 g fat (9% of calories)	11 g fat (27% of calories)
1 g fiber	7 g fiber
2 small blueberry muffins	**2 small oat bran muffins with 2 strips Louis Rich Turkey bacon**
54 g carbohydrates (76% of calories)	55 g carbohydrate (56% of calories)
6 g protein (8% of calories)	12.5 g protein (13% of calories)
5 g fat (16% of calories)	13.8 g fat (31% of calories)
4 g fiber	8.5 g fiber

In Search of the Perfect Breakfast Cereal

You've figured out how to balance your bread or pancakes, but what about that box of cereal? Which ones are best? You could camp out for days in the supermarket aisle reading labels, trying to decide which breakfast cereal to buy. People with diabetes are looking for a few different key items on every cereal label: grams of carbohydrate, grams of soluble fiber, and perhaps calories and sodium. But then you have to compare each figure against about one hundred different cereal selections. This is enough to send even the most motivated person through the exit doors screaming.

Obviously, grams of sugar and carbohydrate need to be considered; some cereals have a lot more added sugar than others, adding a lot of empty calories. Fat and fiber are also an important part of the meal plan. But most cereals aren't that high in fat, with the exception of the traditional granolas. Remember, however, a little fat may actually help people with diabetes control their post-breakfast blood sugar, since fat helps temper the flood of glucose into the bloodstream shortly after a meal containing carbohydrates. So that leaves us with fiber.

Fiber is what separates the special cereals from the masses of boxes on the shelves. Cereals can have anywhere from 1 gram of fiber to 15 grams per serving.

You probably have a pretty good idea of which cereals contribute 1 gram of fiber. But let me help you out on the cereals that contribute 6 grams of fiber or more per serving: Cracklin' Oat Bran, Frosted Mini-Wheats, Fruit & Fibre, Fruitful Bran, Fiber One, Post Bran Flakes, Mueslix Golden Crunch, Multi Bran Chex, Nutri-Grain Golden Wheat with Raisins, All-Bran, Bran Buds, 100% Bran, Quaker 100% Natural Low Fat, Post Raisin Bran, Shredded Wheat 'n Bran, Total Raisin Bran, and regular or instant oatmeal. Do you see a few that you like? I hope so.

Restaurant Tips

Going out for breakfast is one of my favorite things to do. If you like to order eggs, you can ask the cook to make them with egg substitute (many restaurants offer this option). Or, if you like only real eggs, stick to one scrambled egg to keep your dietary cholesterol from skyrocketing (each egg yolk adds 210 milligrams cholesterol to your daily total). Opt for Canadian bacon and fresh fruit as side dishes instead of bacon or sausage if you are trying to cut back on saturated fat (although between the two, bacon will add up to far fewer fat grams than sausage).

If you like oatmeal, it is a good bet because it contributes some soluble fiber. You may want to add some eggs (preferably egg substitute) or a couple of slices of bacon or a sausage link, though, to balance out all that carbohydrate. What about those breakfast potatoes or hash browns? Potatoes are strong carbohydrate contributors, but the way restaurants prepare these potatoes, you are also going to get a stiff dose of cooking oil or shortening—how much depends on the particular cook behind the grill at the greasy spoon you prefer. In general, though, if you stick to $^3/_4$ cup of breakfast potatoes, it will contribute approximately 24 grams carbohydrate and 13 grams fat (220 calories).

MEALTIME TIPS—LUNCH

Sandwiches are one of Americans' favorite lunchtime entrees. Ordering your sandwich on whole wheat will add some fiber, not the soluble fiber that is particularly helpful for people with diabetes, but fiber nonetheless. The glycemic index for whole wheat is virtually the same as for white bread. Shocking but true. If bread is one of your passions, you may want to try switching to an oat bread that you like. If it seems to help, stick with it. The bread I like is Orowheat Light Country Oat Bread. It has 5 grams of fiber, 18 grams of carbohydrate, and 80 calories per 2-slice serving (they are small slices). Even my kids like this bread.

You can make your sandwich with a lean, high-protein filling such as turkey breast or lean ham. If you are making your sandwich at home, you can fix your own chicken or tuna salad using light mayonnaise. You can buy the 50-percent less fat salami and reduced-fat cheeses, too.

You can boost your soluble fiber even more by having your sandwich with a side of three-bean salad or green salad with beans. Eating some fruit with your sandwich is always an option; several common fruits, such as apples, dried apricots, and peaches, have fairly low glycemic indexes.

Restaurant Tips

Choose sandwiches made with lean roast beef, lean ham, or turkey breast. Order the sandwich with ketchup, barbecue sauce, or mustard instead of mayonnaise (unless they have reduced-fat mayonnaise), thousand island dressing, or "secret" or tartar sauce. The same goes for dressing burgers and chicken and fish sandwiches. Just eliminating the mayonnaise or creamy sauce can cut 15 grams of fat off the top. Chances are you are already getting plenty of fat and protein to help balance your carbohydrates from whatever is in between the bun. You probably don't need the fat from the sauce too.

If you tend to go to the same fast-food chains or restaurants, check out their nutritional analysis brochure or chart, which should be posted in the restaurant (and see the nutritional information offered in this book). This information can help you figure out which items best fit into your eating plan.

Take a look at the sandwich selections profiled below:

1.   3 ounces sliced smokey turkey breast and $1/4$ avocado on two slices of mixed-grain bread, with mustard; $1/3$ cup of three-bean salad; 8 ounces of apple juice (459 calories, 58 g carbohydrate [50% of calories], 27 g protein [22% of calories], 14.5 g fat [28% of calories], 7 g fiber)

2.   3 ounces lean ham and 1 ounce reduced fat cheese on a sourdough bun, with 1 tablespoon light mayonnaise, a green salad with $1/3$ cup kidney beans and light dressing or a bowl of soup with beans (535 calories, 51 g carbohydrate [38% of calories], 37.8 g protein [28% of calories], 20.5 g fat [34% of calories], 9.5 g fiber)

MEALTIME TIPS—DINNER

Take it off. Take it all off! What are we talking about? Chicken skin, of course. Removing the skin will save you half the fat calories. When ordering or buying steak, select the leaner cuts such as London broil, chateaubriand, or filet mignon. You can use homemade or commercial marinades to help tenderize the tougher steaks. Trim the fat you see on your steak or meat with your knife. In a restaurant, you can order the petite servings to keep your serving sizes moderate

Probably your greatest challenge at evening meals is keeping your serving sizes moderate. Americans tend to make dinner, their last meal of the day, their heaviest and largest. Try to stick closely to your eating plan, meeting your grams of carbohydrate as closely as possible. This might mean measuring your rice or pasta from time to time to make sure your carbohydrate count is accurate.

If you feel too hungry at bedtime, talk to your health care team or dietitian for help in adjusting your medication or eating plan (they might add a small evening snack) so things work out better at bedtime. Remember the section on free foods earlier in this chapter, too.

For more mealtime tips for dinner and more tips to help you eat out, see the next section on "solving the dining-out dilemna."

SOLVING THE DINING-OUT DILEMMA

Fast Food Is a Part of Life

A week doesn't go by where my family doesn't end up ordering at least one lunch or dinner from a fast-food chain. After all, pizza is one of our favorite foods—with cheeseburgers, Mexican food, and chicken and fish sandwiches following close behind. So with the convenience and cost of fast food, there is almost no reason not to go to many of these fast-food chains every now and then. That is, unless you are watching your calories, fiber and fat grams, and—oh yes—sodium.

In general, fast food is high in fat, sodium, and calories (sometimes also high in saturated fat and cholesterol) while being very low in fiber—a particularly bad combination for those with diabetes.

So what's a fast-food lover to do? Make informed selections. Thumb through the list of better fast-food choices in the table below and try to find at least one that you would like at each of the fast-food chains you tend to visit. Next time, try this item, counting it into your C-F-F (carbohydrate, fat, and fiber) eating plan. You will probably need to B.Y.O.F. (bring your own fiber), though. You can supplement your fast-food meal with some high-fiber foods from home (carrot or asparagus sticks, apple or orange wedges, broccoli or cauliflower stems) or make a point to add beans to a green salad at the salad bar.

It's easy to add fiber to pizza—just order a vegetarian pizza. Tell them to load on the mushrooms, peppers, onions, artichoke hearts, zucchini, and so forth. Granted, this may be difficult for professed pepperoni pizza eaters, but for me it's a piece of (carrot) cake!

Better Fast-Food Choices for Your C-F-F Counting Plan

The following fast-food items have 40 percent or fewer calories from fat, unless preceded by an asterisk (*). The asterisked items were included because they are low in grams of fat or have other redeeming qualities (i.e., contain vegetables).

Burger King

	Calories	Carbo-hydrate (g)	Fat (g)	Calories from fat (%)	Fiber (g)	Sodium (mg)	Choles-terol (mg)
Sandwiches							
Whopper without mayonnaise	430	45	16.0	33	3.0	710	70
hamburger	330	28	15.0	41	1.0	530	55
BK Big Fish	520	56	22.0	38	3.0	760	75
BK Broiler (chicken)	340	41	6.0	16	2.0	320	60
chicken sandwich	500	54	20.0	36	2.0	1,240	40

	Cal- ories	Carbo- hydrate (g)	Fat (g)	Calories from fat (%)	Fiber (g)	Sodium (mg)	Choles- terol (mg)
Salads							
*broiled chicken salad with reduced-calorie Italian dressing	215	10	10.5	44	3.0	160	60
*garden salad with reduced-calorie Italian dressing	115	10	5.5	43	3.0	160	15

Boston Market (800-365-7000)

Boston Market has over one thousand stores in all but fifteen states.

	Cal- ories	Carbo- hydrate (g)	Fat (g)	Calories from fat (%)	Fiber (g)	Sodium (mg)	Choles- terol (mg)
Entrees							
1/4 white meat chicken, no skin or wing	160	0	3.5	20	0	350	95
*1/4 dark meat chicken, no skin	210	1.0	10.0	43	0	320	150
skinless rotisserie turkey breast, 5 oz.	170	1.0	1.0	5	0	850	100
ham with cinnamon apples, 8 oz.	350	335	13.0	33	2.0	1750	75
*meat loaf and chunky tomato sauce, 8 oz.	370	22	18.0	44	2.0	1170	120
*Original Chicken Pot Pie, 1	750	78	34.0	41	6.0	2380	115
Soups, Salads, and Sandwiches							
*Caesar salad, no dressing	240	14	13.0	49	3.0	780	25
chicken soup	80	4.0	3.0	34	1.0	470	25
chicken sandwich, no sauce or cheese	430	61	3.5	8	5.0	860	95
turkey sandwich, no sauce or cheese	400	61	3.5	8	4.0	1070	60
ham sandwich, no cheese or sauce	450	66	9.0	18	4.0	1600	45
meat loaf sandwich, no cheese	690	86	21.0	27	6.0	1610	120

(continued)

	Cal- ories	Carbo- hydrate (g)	Fat (g)	Calories from fat (%)	Fiber (g)	Sodium (mg)	Choles- terol (mg)
ham and turkey club sandwich, no cheese or sauce	430	64	6.0	13	4.0	1330	55
Side Dishes (³/₄ cup unless otherwise noted)							
steamed vegetables	35	7	0.5	13	3.0	35	0
new potatoes	140	25	3.0	19	2.0	100	0
buttered corn	190	39	4.0	19	4.0	130	0
rice pilaf, ²/₃ cup	180	32	5.0	25	2.0	600	0
stuffing	310	44	12.0	35	3.0	1140	0
butternut squash	160	25	6.0	34	3.0	580	15
macaroni and cheese	280	36	10.0	32	1.0	760	20
BBQ baked beans	330	53	9.0	25	9.0	630	10
hot cinnamon apples	250	56	4.5	16	3.0	45	0
fruit salad	70	17	0.5	6	2.0	10	0
*Mediterranean pasta salad	170	16	10.0	53	2.0	490	10
cranberry relish, ¹/₈ cup	61	14	1.0	15	1.0	1	0
corn bread, 1 loaf	200	33	6.0	27	1.0	390	25

Domino's Pizza (313-930-3030)

	Cal- ories	Carbo- hydrate (g)	Fat (g)	Calories from fat (%)	Fiber (g)	Sodium (mg)	Choles- terol (mg)
Breadsticks, 1 piece	78	11	3.5	40	—	158	—
garden salad, small, with light Italian dressing	42	6.0	1.3	28	2.0	14	0
garden salad, large, with light Italian dressing	59	10	1.5	23	3.0	26	0
Pizza (14-inch large), hand-tossed, cheese (2 of 12 slices)	319	44	10.0	28	2.0	622	18

Note: Domino's deep-dish pizza has twice the fat of the thin crust or hand-tossed pizza. Ordering pepperoni pizza will add 55 calories, 5 grams of fat (2 grams saturated fat), and 11 mg cholesterol per serving.

Hardee's (800-564-2733)

Breakfast

	Cal- ories	Carbo- hydrate (g)	Fat (g)	Calories from fat (%)	Fiber (g)	Sodium (mg)	Choles- terol (mg)
apple cinnamon 'n' raisin biscuit	200	30	8.0	36	N/A	350	0
three pancakes	280	56	2.0	6	N/A	890	15

	Cal-ories	Carbo-hydrate (g)	Fat (g)	Calories from fat (%)	Fiber (g)	Sodium (mg)	Choles-terol (mg)
Sandwiches							
hamburger	270	29	11.0	37	N/A	670	35
chicken fillet	480	54	18.0	34	N/A	1280	55
grilled chicken	350	38	11.0	28	N/A	950	65
hot ham 'n' cheese	310	34	12.0	35	N/A	1410	50
fried chicken breast	370	29	15.0	36	N/A	1190	75
Other							
mashed potatoes and gravy	90	17	~1.0	<10	N/A	590	0
baked beans	170	32	1.0	5	N/A	600	0
grilled chicken salad (no dressing)	150	11	3.0	18	N/A	610	60
French fries, small	240	33	10.0	38	N/A	100	0

Jack-in-the-Box (800-207-5225)

	Cal-ories	Carbo-hydrate (g)	Fat (g)	Calories from fat (%)	Fiber (g)	Sodium (mg)	Choles-terol (mg)
Breakfast							
Breakfast Jack	300	30	12.0	36	0	890	185
Pancake Platter	400	59	12.0	27	3.0	980	30
Pancake syrup	120	30	0.0	0	0	5.0	0
Sandwiches							
Chicken Fajita Pita	290	29	8.0	25	3.0	700	35
Chicken Sandwich	400	38	18.0	40	0	1290	45
Grilled Chicken Fillet	430	36	19.0	40	0	1070	65
Hamburger	280	31	11.0	35	0	470	25
Other							
Garden Chicken Salad	200	8	9.0	40	3.0	420	65
*Side Salad	70	3	4.0	51	2.0	80	10
*Side Salad with Low-cal Italian dressing and croutons	145	13	7.5	46	2.0	855	10

(continued)

	Cal- ories	Carbo- hydrate (g)	Fat (g)	Calories from fat (%)	Fiber (g)	Sodium (mg)	Choles- terol (mg)
Chicken Teriyaki Bowl, no soy sauce	580	115	1.5	2	6.0	1220	30

Note: Many people with diabetes may not do well with this item. Although it contains a nice chunk of fiber, it is very high in carbohydrate grams, while being very low in fat and prohibitively high in sodium, even without the soy sauce.

Chicken Strips, 4	290	18	13.0	40	0	700	50
Barbecue Dipping Sauce	45	11	0.0	0	0	300	0
Sweet & Sour Dipping Sauce	40	11	0.0	0	0	160	0

KFC (Public Affairs Dept., P.O. Box 32070, Louisville, KY 40232)

Tender Roast Chicken Breast w/o skin	169	1.0	4.0	21	0	797	112
Tender Roast Breast with skin	251	1.0	11.0	39	0	830	151
Original Recipe chicken sandwich	497	45.5	22.5	40	3.0	1213	52
barbecue chicken sandwich	256	28	8.0	28	2.0	782	57
corn on the cob	190	34	3.0	14	4.0	20	0
BBQ baked beans	190	33	3.0	14	6.0	760	5
red beans and rice	130	21	3.0	21	3.0	360	5
Garden rice	120	23	1.5	11	1.0	890	0
*mashed potatoes with gravy	120	17	6.0	45	2.0	440	<1
*Mean Greens	70	11	3.0	53	5.0	360	5
*Tender Roast Thigh without skin	106	<1	5.5	47	0	312	84

Note: An Original Recipe breast contains 24 grams of fat, an Extra Tasty Crispy breast contains 28 grams, and a Hot and Spicy breast has 35 grams.

Long John Silver's (800-880-FISH)

Flavorbaked Fish, 1	90	1.0	2.5	25	0	320	35
Flavorbaked Chicken (2.6 ounces)	110	<1	13.0	25	<1	600	55

Sandwiches

Batter-Dipped Fish (no sauce)	320	40	13.0	37	6.0	800	30
Flavorbaked Fish	320	28	14.0	39	2.0	930	55

	Cal- ories	Carbo- hydrate (g)	Fat (g)	Calories from fat (%)	Fiber (g)	Sodium (mg)	Choles- terol (mg)
Flavorbaked Chicken	290	27	10.0	31	2.0	970	60
Hushpuppy, 2 pieces	120	18	5.0	38	0	25	0
Corn Cobbette without							
butter	80	19	0.5	6	0	0	0
Rice Pilaf	140	26	3.0	19	3.0	260	0

McDonald's (630-623-FOOD)

hamburger	270	34	10.0	33	2.0	530	30
cheeseburger	320	35	14.0	39	2.0	770	45
Fish Filet Deluxe							
without tartar sauce	437	59	13.0	27	5.0	926	42
Crispy Chicken							
Deluxe without mayo	389	47	11.0	25	4.0	1031	45
Grilled Chicken Deluxe							
with 1 pkg. honey							
mustard	380	45	10.5	25	4.0	1055	60
with 1 pkg. barbecue							
sauce	375	52	6.0	14	4.0	1220	50
Fajita Chicken Salad							
with 1 pkg. Lite Vinai-							
grette Dressing	210	18	8.0	34	3.0	640	65
Egg McMuffin	290	27	13.0	40	1.0	730	235
Hot Cakes (plain)	310	53	7.0	20	2.0	610	15
Hot Cakes plus syrup							
and 2 pats margarine	580	100	16.0	25	2.0	760	15

Pizza Hut (800-948-8488)

2 slices of medium pizza							
hand-tossed cheese	470	59	14.0	27	4.0	1242	50
hand-tossed ham	426	58	10.0	21	4.0	1314	42
hand-tossed pepperoni	476	58	16.0	30	4.0	1378	48
hand-tossed veggie							
lover's	432	60	12.0	25	6.0	1264	34
2 slices cheese Bigfoot	372	50	12.0	29	4.0	1050	32

Round Table Pizza (800-753-2825)

Salute Veggie (2 slices							
of a large thin pizza)	280	38	9.0	29	N/A	N/A	20

(continued)

	Cal-ories	Carbo-hydrate (g)	Fat (g)	Calories from fat (%)	Fiber (g)	Sodium (mg)	Choles-terol (mg)
Salute Cashew Chicken (2 slices of a large thin pizza)	280	40	8.0	26	N/A	N/A	30
Gourmet Veggie	320	38	14.0	39	N/A	N/A	30
Gourmet Chicken & garlic (2 slices of a large thin pizza)	340	34	14.0	37	N/A	N/A	50

Taco Bell (800-822-6235)

Double Decker Taco	340	37	15.0	40	8.0	700	30
Steak Soft Taco	200	18	7.0	31	1.0	500	25
Bean Burrito	380	55	12.0	28	12	1140	10
Burrito Supreme	440	50	18.0	37	8.0	1220	45
7-Layer Burrito	540	65	24.0	40	14	1310	25
Chili Cheese Burrito	330	37	13.0	35	4.0	880	35
*Tostada	300	31	14.0	42	11	700	15
Light Chicken Burrito	310	41	8.0	23	3.0	980	25
Light Chicken Burrito Supreme	430	52	13.0	27	3.0	1410	55
Light Chicken Soft Taco	180	21	5.0	25	2.0	660	25
*Pintos 'n Cheese	190	18	8.0	43	10	690	15

Wendy's (510-937-7269)

Sandwiches

Breaded chicken with ketchup, no mayo	390	45	13.0	30	2.0	790	55
Chicken club with catsup, no mayo	460	46	18.0	35	2.0	1040	70
Grilled chicken with reduced-calorie honey mustard	290	35	7.0	22	2.0	720	55
Jr. Hamburger	270	34	9.0	30	2.0	600	35
Jr. Cheeseburger	320	34	13.0	37	2.0	770	45
Plain Single (^{1}/4-lb. patty plus bun)	350	31	15.0	39	2.0	510	70
Broccoli & Cheese Potato	460	79	14.0	27	9.0	440	0
Sour Cream & Chives Potato	380	74	6.0	14	8.0	40	15

	Cal- ories	Carbo- hydrate (g)	Fat (g)	Calories from fat (%)	Fiber (g)	Sodium (mg)	Choles- terol (mg)
Chili, small	190	20	6.0	28	5.0	670	40
Chili, large	290	31	9.0	28	7.0	1000	60
*Grilled chicken salad plus 2 Tb. reduced-fat ranch	260	12	13.0	45	4.0	970	60
Deluxe garden salad plus 2 Tb. reduced-fat ranch	170	12	11.0	58	4.0	600	10

The Art of Dining When You've Got Diabetes

For business or for pleasure, eating out in restaurants is a must. There is no reason why people with diabetes can't comfortably and successfully eat many of their meals in restaurants. As I see it, there are three tricks to eating out when you have diabetes:

Trick #1: Order foods that will be more likely to encourage normal blood glucose levels.

Trick #2: Eat the right amounts of those foods to encourage normal blood glucose levels.

Trick #3: Time your meals correctly with medication such as diabetes pills or insulin.

Master these three tricks and you will most likely have mastered the art of dining when you've got diabetes. In order to help you with Trick #1, see the table on page 146, listing the fifteen most commonly ordered restaurant items, their approximate nutritional analysis, and suggestions. Refer also to the mealtime tips section earlier in this chapter. Finally, don't be afraid to ask if food can be cooked or served differently from what's on the menu. Restaurants are in the business of keeping their customers happy, or at least they should be.

Usually, it is no problem to ask that your fish be grilled instead of fried or that your sandwich be served with mustard instead of mayonnaise. Often, you can even substitute healthier side dishes for the ones that normally come with your entrée. You can ask for a baked potato instead of french fries, a green salad instead of coleslaw, or fresh vegetables instead of potato salad. One of my favorite restaurant requests is to ask if sauces or salad dressings can be served "on the side." This way *you* control the amount added to your meal. For example, I love ordering Chinese chicken salad in restaurants, but I know the dressing is usually half oil. If I ask for the dressing on the side, I can pour two tablespoons over the top and know that I haven't done too much damage at the meal.

To tackle Trick #2, review the portion control section in chapter 5 and the following restaurant tips:

- Order an appetizer or two as a main meal or split a main dish with your dining companion.
- Enjoy noncaloric beverages such as mineral water, coffee, or tea, and/or enjoy a green salad or broth-based soup to help fill you up a little before the entrée comes.
- Look forward to leftovers. Right off the bat, set aside a portion of your dinner to be enjoyed all over again at home—tomorrow.
- Avoid buffet restaurants, especially if you know you can't resist eating too much, either because you love the food or because you want to get your money's worth.

Timing your medication correctly with your restaurant meal, Trick #3, is challenging, because you rarely control how long the wait for a table is, how good the service is, and how quickly the food gets to the table. You may want to take the pills or insulin after you get to the restaurant in case your meal is delayed or the wait for a table is longer than expected. If you are in a situation where you have to eat *earlier* than usual, stick with an appetizer, or just part of a meal, and save the rest for later. If you are in a situation where you have to eat *later* than usual, eat a snack when you would normally eat your meal. If you have already taken your medication only to discover the wait for your meal is longer than expected, order a quick appetizer or munch on pretzels to tide you over. It's a good idea to test you blood sugar more often than you normally would when you are eating out to prevent high and low blood glucose levels.

Most Ordered Menu Items

The following nutrition information is an approximation, based on data from the *Food Processor* nutritional analysis computer program.

	Calories	Carbohydrate (g)	Fat (g)	Calories from fat (%)	Fiber (g)	Sodium* (mg)	Cholesterol (mg)
1. Hamburger or Cheeseburger							
¹/₄-lb. patty plus bun	377	23	19.0	46	1.0	331	86
¹/₄-lb. patty plus bun plus 1 oz. cheese	489	23	28.0	52	1.0	502	113
mayo, 1 Tb.	99		11.0			78	8
ketchup, 1 Tb.	16	4.0	0.0	0	0	182	0
mustard, 1.5 tsp.	6	0.5	0.5	48	0	98	0
BBQ sauce, 1 Tb.	25	5.5	0.0	0	0	225	0
2. Salads (per cup)							
chef-type salad	178	3.0	10.5	54	N/A	495	93
spinach salad, no dressing	89	10	4.0	39	1.5	157	61
creamy salad dressing	55	1	5.5			100	6
3. French Fries							
French fries, 1 cup	180	23	9.5	46	2.0	123	0
4. Steak or Roast Beef							
5 oz. T-bone, trimmed of visible fat, grilled	304	0	15.0	45	0	93	113
3 oz. roast beef, trimmed of visible fat	170	0	6.0	34	0	43	82
5. Pizza (see Fast-Food Choices for Your C-F-F Counting Plan)							
6. Baked Whole Potatoes							
long potato with skin	220	50	0.0	1	5.0	16	0
medium potato with skin	133	30	0.0	1	3.0	10	0
1 pat (tsp.) butter	34	0	4.0	100	0	39	10
1 Tb. sour cream	31	1.0	3.0	86	0	8	6

7. Fish (Of course there are many types of fish, each one having a different nutritional breakdown, but here are a few of the more popular items.)

	Calories	Carbohydrate (g)	Fat (g)	Calories from fat (%)	Fiber (g)	Sodium* (mg)	Cholesterol (mg)
1 piece swordfish, 3¹/₂ oz., broiled	164	0	5.5	31	0	122	53
fried fish fillet, 3 oz.	211	15.5	13.0	50	0	484	31

*Sodium values, in some cases, do not reflect any extra salt that may be added by restaurants.

(continued)

	Cal- ories	Carbo- hydrate (g)	Fat (g)	Calories from fat (%)	Fiber (g)	Sodium* (mg)	Choles- terol (mg)
8. Fried Chicken							
breast	410	18	26.0	59	4.0	600	85
thigh	260	10	18.0	62	2.0	540	65
9. Soup, 1 cup							
cream of broccoli	234	16	16.0	59	2.0	788	23
minestrone	127	21	3.0	20	2.0	864	5
10. Ice Cream							
1/2 cup rich ice cream	178	17	12.0	58	0	41	45
11. Grilled or Broiled Chicken							
breast, no skin	142	0	3.0	21	0	73	64
breast, with skin	193	0	7.5	37	0	70	82
thigh, no skin	109	0	5.5	49	0	46	49
thigh, with skin	153	0	9.6	58	0	52	58
12. Rice, 1 cup							
steamed	267	58	0.5	2	1.0	2.0	0
fried rice	264	34	12.0	40	1.0	286	42
rice pilaf	268	46	7.0	23	1.0	754	0
Spanish rice	216	41	4.0	16	1.0	324	0
13. Ham, Bacon, or Sausage							
ham, 2 oz.	89	0	3.0	33	0	752	31
bacon strips, 2 small	73	0	6.0	78	0	202	11
Canadian bacon, 2 slices							
(50 g)	90	0	4.0	43	0	727	27
2 sausage links (50 g)	170	0	15.0	78	0	414	40
14. Shrimp or Lobster							
lobster tail (125 g)	145	2.0	4.0	24	0	777	95
1 Tb. butter	102	0	11.5	100	0	117	31
tiger prawns, breaded							
and fried, 3 oz.	206	10	10.5	46	0	292	150
tiger prawns, steamed	84	0	1.0	11	0	190	165

15. Chicken Sandwich (see Fast-Food Choices for Your C-F-F Counting Plan)

	Cal- ories	Carbo- hydrate (g)	Fat (g)	Calories from fat (%)	Fiber (g)	Sodium* (mg)	Choles- terol (mg)
Foods That People Are Ordering More Frequently Than Before							
Frozen Yogurt, 1 cup							
vanilla or fruit	203	37	2.6	11	0	118	10
chocolate	230	36	8.0	32	3.0	141	7
Asian Foods, 1 cup							
cashew chicken	310	15	21.0	58	3.0	990	33
broccoli beef	202	7.0	12.5	55	3.0	753	34
fried tofu and vegetables	125	8.0	9.0	59	3.0	900	0
Tacos or Taco Salad							
beef taco, small	190	15	11.0	52	2.0	410	20
beef taco, large	369	27	20.0	49	N/A	802	56
chicken soft taco	223	20	10.0	40	N/A	553	58
taco salad, salsa, and shell	940	70	60.0	56	11	1,771	88
Turkey, 3 oz.							
roasted turkey, combination light and dark meat	145	0	4.0	28	0	60	64
Pasta or Pasta Salad							
Italian pasta salad, 1 cup	348	33	21.0	55	5.0	864	0
Spaghetti with meat sauce, 1¹/2 cups	498	58	17.0	32	11	1514	112
1 cup egg noodles plus ¹/2 cup white sauce	390	50	16.0	37	2.5	196	67
1 cup egg noodles plus ¹/4 cup pesto	524	44	31.0	53	3.0	433	70
Top Breakfast Items							
Eggs and Omelets 1 scrambled egg	101	1.0	7.0	67	0	171	215
1 scrambled egg (egg substitute plus 1 tsp. margarine)	65	1.0	4.0	55	0	135	0

(continued)

	Cal-ories	Carbo-hydrate (g)	Fat (g)	Calories from fat (%)	Fiber (g)	Sodium* (mg)	Choles-terol (mg)
2 eggs, ham and cheese omelet	284	2.0	22.0	70	0	736	462
ham and cheese omelet w/egg substitute	259	2.0	15.0	54	0	740	52
Muffins							
blueberry, 1 small (45 g)	131	18	5.0	35	1.0	198	18
bran, 1 small (45 g)	130	19	6.0	37	3.0	265	16
Bagels							
plain, 1	195	38	1.0	5	2.0	379	0
whole wheat, 1	145	31	1.0	4	5.0	270	0
cream cheese, 2 Tb.	97	1.0	10.0	88	0	82	31

*Sodium values, in some cases, do not reflect any extra salt that may be added by restaurants.

TAKE IT ONE STEP AT A TIME

Having diabetes can feel as if you are learning to walk (or eat) all over again. You are learning good habits and, very likely, trying to change some bad ones. You are being asked to write down what you eat, and you are being asked to keep track of calories, carbohydrates, fat, fiber, and blood sugar levels. It may seem that whim and spontaneity are gone forever from mealtime.

Patience. Take it one step at a time. You are more likely to make it down the stairs in one piece if you do. If you try to fly down the staircase, going down too many steps at once, you may end up at the bottom of the stairs, with a bruised hip (or ego) and a full dose of frustration.

Changing too many habits too soon can be overwhelming, even on a good day. Instead, set yourself up for success. Tackle the easiest habit first. Once you've got one change under your belt, perhaps the next might not seem as bad. If you don't know which behavior or goal you should work on first, ask you health care team to help you prioritize them. Setting a realistic goal and allowing a reasonable amount of time to accomplish it increases the likeli-hood of long-term success.

In order for these changes or new behaviors to last a lifetime, they need to be integrated into your lifestyle. And remember, practice makes perfect.

Every day you practice your new habit or behavior, the next day should get a little easier.

Praising yourself for your accomplishments and finding support and reinforcement from friends, family, and others with diabetes are also important. If you don't have this support in your life right now, you may need to find it. There are diabetes support groups for people with diabetes all over the country that generally meet monthly. If you have a health care team that isn't offering you adequate support, change to one that does—if you can. Not only do you deserve this support, your diabetes management is more likely to be successful if you have it in your life.

DIABETIC BY MARRIAGE

Given that I'm married to a Magee, I've always gotten a kick out of those T-shirts that say IRISH BY MARRIAGE. After writing this book and speaking with many spouses of people with diabetes, I've thought of another T-shirt slogan: DIABETIC BY MARRIAGE.

Your spouse may sometimes feel as if she (yes, I know it can be *he* as well) has diabetes by osmosis. She reads books and cookbooks along with you; she has changed the way she prepares many foods. She may go with you to support groups or meetings. She may even be counting carbohydrate, fat, and fiber grams to help you follow your eating plan as closely as possible. Take a moment to pat your spouse on the back; her support and involvement in your eating plan are crucial to your success. According to a study of 254 married men with high cholesterol levels, those whose wives supported their dietary changes were more likely to maintain a low-fat diet over the long run. Twenty-four months after an eight-week nutrition class, 51 percent of the men with the most spousal support met their dietary goals, compared to 28 percent of those with the least support. You're in this together.

7

SUPERMARKET SCORE CARD—THE BEST BETS FOR DISCRIMINATING PEOPLE WITH DIABETES

"But does it taste good?" is my conditioned response to the news that a fat-free or sugar-free product has just hit the market. I always try these products with as open a mind as I can muster. Sometimes I'm pleasantly surprised, but more often than not, I end up throwing it out. I asked a group of people with diabetes to help me taste-test many of the less-sugar, no-sugar, and less-fat products on the market. The results are described here, along with a nutritional assessment of the top-rated products.

DOES NO SUGAR MEAN BAD FLAVOR?

You're shopping as you do every week, minding your own business, when suddenly out jumps a red-and-white label reading "no sugar added" from a carton of ice cream or yogurt or a package of cookies. Immediately your heart starts pumping, your mind starts racing. Could this really be something I can eat and enjoy? So you buy it. Only it tastes terrible, and you end up throwing the product away along with the three dollars it took to try it. Sound familiar?

Do you try the next no-sugar product that comes along? Maybe. Probably. Because you know from experience that every now and then you hit the jackpot. Sometimes you find a product you actually like. Finding those surprisingly good products was the purpose of this chapter.

I'll tell you which products the tasters liked and which ones they threw away in disgust. I'll tell you which ones score high or low on the nutrition index for fat, carbohydrate, calories, and sodium. My hope is to save you time and money and feelings of hopelessness when you've thrown out your fifth new product in a row.

I had to research the physiology and science of tastes and flavors when I wrote a book called *Taste vs. Fat: Rating the Low-Fat and Fat-Free Foods* (1997). So it is from experience that I can tell you that all taste buds are *not* created equal. Some are more sensitive than others to differences in fat, sugar, or sodium. Some are more sensitive to aftertastes and bitterness. Such individuality is another reason why I felt it was important to have a large group of people test each product.

The primary taste issue with no-sugar products is whether or not there is a strong aftertaste, since most of these products use large quantities of artificial sweeteners. Also, some products contain sugar alcohols—sorbitol or mannitol—which in medium to large amounts can give you diarrhea. So these additives are also noted in the tables that follow.

Of course, you'll find the calories and grams of protein, carbohydrates, sugar, fat, and fiber, and milligrams of sodium and cholesterol listed for each of these products as well.

READING LABELS

If you are going to read one label on the package, make it the *Nutrition Facts* label. Sure the list of ingredients is interesting and sometimes helpful (ingredients in packaged foods are listed by *weight* from the most to least), but the Nutrition Facts label is the label that lists the calories, grams of carbohydrate, fat, and fiber per serving.

Ingredient lists are particularly helpful for people who are sensitive or allergic to certain ingredients. For example, if you have a problem with too much sorbitol or mannitol, etc., you'll want to read the label to see if that product contains any sugar alcohols.

Once you find the Nutrition Facts label of a food product, what do you look for?

- Look at the serving size listed. Ask yourself, "is this more or less than the amount I normally eat?" "Is it more or less than the amount listed in my eating plan?" If you eat two times more than the amount listed, you'll need to double the calories and grams of carbohydrate, fat, and fiber in your mealtime calculations.

- Look at the nutrients that you are most interested in, such as total grams of carbohydrate and fat, and possibly grams of saturated fat, and milligrams of cholesterol and sodium. You will find these nutrients and numbers on the left-hand side of the Nutrition Facts label. Typically serving size is listed first, then you'll see calories, total fat, saturated fat, cholesterol, sodium, then finally total carbohydrate, dietary fiber, grams of sugar, and protein.

On the right side of the Nutrition Facts label you will find the % Daily Value listed. This is similar to the Recommended Daily Allowances (RDA) of years past. The % Daily Value on the food label tells you how much of the Daily Values you use up when you eat one serving of this particular food item if following a 2,000 calorie eating plan.

For example, it is recommended that people eat 30 percent calories or fewer from fat; 30 percent of 2,000 calories is 65 grams of fat per day. So, if a food product contains 3 grams of fat per serving, the % Daily Value column will read 5%, because 3 grams of fat is 5% of 65 grams.

If this confuses you, you are not alone. My advice is to concentrate on the *left* portion of the Nutrition Facts label. As someone with diabetes you have hopefully already worked out a personalized eating plan with your dietitian or diabetes educator with a target number of calories, grams of carbohydrate, and so on. This is the plan you need to follow closely. And the numbers to the left of the Nutrition Facts label will help you count your calories and grams of carbohydrate, fat, and fiber to help you follow that personal eating plan.

Nutrition Facts	
Serving Size 1/2 Cup (63g)	
Servings Per Container 16	
Amount Per Serving	
Calories 130	Calories from Fat 50
	% Daily Value*
Total Fat 5g	**8%**
Saturated Fat 3g	**15%**
Cholesterol 15mg	**6%**
Sodium 55mg	**2%**
Total Carbohydrate 19g	**6%**
Dietary Fiber 0g	**0%**
Sugars 17g	
Protein 2g	

This sample label for a popular light ice cream shows how all the data are listed.

RATING THE "NO-SUGAR" AND "LESS-SUGAR" PRODUCTS FOR TASTE AND NUTRITION

There are three types of no-sugar products in the supermarkets: (1) no-sugar products with just as much fat as the regular product, (2) no-sugar products that also have reduced or eliminated the fat, and (3) no-sugar products that didn't have any fat to begin with. Products like juice popsicles, jams, and hard candy would be in the last category.

Fat plays a pivotal role in the palatability of certain foods such as dairy, frozen desserts, meat, and chocolate products. When you reduce or eliminate the fat in certain foods, you often change the texture and reduce the sensory quality of the food. In other words, it doesn't taste as good. To help compensate for this loss of taste sensation and texture, manufacturers often replace some or all of the fat with a carbohydrate. So don't be surprised to find some reduced-fat or fat-free products to be *higher* in total grams of carbohydrate (sodium also tends to increase).

This is one nutritional reason why the sugar-free products that still have some fat tend to be the better options for people with diabetes. Not only do they taste better than the sugar-free or fat-free options, they also tend to have fewer grams of carbohydrate per serving. Take sugar-free ice cream as one example. The sugar-free and fat-free ice creams I tried tasted terrible, and they also contained 3 more grams of carbohydrate per $1/2$-cup serving. The 3 grams of fat that the sugar-free (reduced-fat) ice cream contained was well worth it—it tasted much better than the fat-free. And after all, we are talking about 3 grams of fat, not 30! (But keep in mind the serving size.)

NO SUGAR ADDED

Chocolate Milk Powder

Nestlé's Quik No Sugar Added (with NutraSweet)

Serving	Calories	Fat (g)	Saturated Fat (g)	Total Carbohydrate (g)	Sugar (g)
2 Tb.	40	1	.5	7	1

Chocolate milk is a popular drink in my house, so it was our pleasure to try the new Nestlé Quik No Sugar Added chocolate milk powder. We all love it. My husband was a little skeptical when he heard it had no sugar added, but even he liked it when it was mixed with milk. Because the 1 gram of sugar it contains per serving is from lactose (milk sugar), the product can still be classified as no sugar added. Recall that lactose has about half the glycemic index of glucose.

Flavored Coffee

I've spoken with quite a few coffee lovers with diabetes who love these sugar-free flavored coffees. If you like instant coffee, you'll probably like these.

French Vanilla Cafe Sugar Free* Fat Free (General Foods International Coffees)

Serving	Calories	Fat (g)	Saturated Fat (g)	Total Carbohydrate (g)	Sugar (g)
1¹/₃ Tb.	25	0	0	5	0

*Contains NutraSweet.

Cafe Vienna Sugar Free* Fat Free (General Foods International Coffees)

Serving	Calories	Fat (g)	Saturated Fat (g)	Total Carbohydrate (g)	Sugar (g)
1¹/₃ Tb.	30	1.5	.5	3	0

*Contains NutraSweet.

Hot Cocoa

Quite a few tasters thought both brands of No Sugar Added Hot Cocoa Mix were fine, as far as instant cocoa goes.

Carnation No Sugar Added Hot Cocoa Mix

Serving	Calories	Fat (g)	Saturated Fat (g)	Total Carbohydrate (g)	Sugar (g)
1 packet	50	0	0	8	7

The 7 grams of sugar are from the lactose (milk sugar) present in nonfat dry milk, which is the first ingredient. NutraSweet is used as the sweetener.

Swiss Miss No Sugar Added Hot Cocoa Mix

Serving	Calories	Fat (g)	Saturated Fat (g)	Total Carbohydrate (g)	Sugar (g)
1 packet	50	0	0	10	7

The 7 grams of sugar are from the lactose (milk sugar) present in the sweet dairy whey and nonfat dry milk (the first and second ingredients). NutraSweet is used as the sweetener.

Candy

While most of the following sugar-free candies tasted similar to the regular versions, their carbohydrate grams per serving were also similar. So, if you are counting grams of carbohydrate, there is little point in purchasing these alternative candies.

Gummy Bears

	Serving	Calories	Total Carbohydrate (g)
Estee Sugar Free Gummy Bears	17 (41 g)	100	30
Regular Gummy Bears	14 (41 g)	130	29

The sugar-free gummy bears are going to save you 30 calories per serving, but they contain almost the same amount of carbohydrate compared to the regular gummy bears. I prefer the taste and texture of the regular gummy bears, and so did most of my tasters.

Peppermint Candy

	Serving	Calories	Total Carbohydrate (g)
Estee Sugar Free Peppermint Swirls	3 (14 g)	60	14
Brach's Star Brites (regular)	3 (15 g)	60	15

The sugar-free peppermint candies were liked by most tasters. However, as you can see, they contain just as many calories and almost the same amount of carbohydrates as the Brach's peppermint candies.

Butterscotch Candy

	Serving	Calories	Total Carbohydrate (g)
Estee Sugar Free Butterscotch	3 (18 g)	75	18
Farley's Butter Toffee	3 (16 g)	70	14

The sugar-free butterscotch candies tasted great. Most tasters really liked them. They aren't going to save you any calories or grams of carbohydrate though.

Cookies

	Serving	Calories (g)	Total Carbohydrate (g)	Fat
Estee Fructose Sweetened Sandwich Cookies	3 (34 g)	160	24	6
Estee Sugar-Free Creme Wafers, Lemon	5 (33 g)	160	22	8

Compare to:

	Serving	Calories (g)	Total Carbohydrate (g)	Fat
Reduced Fat Oreo	3 (32 g)	130	25	3.5
Mother's Checkerboard Wafers	8 (30 g)	150	20	8

This is a perfect example of products that may not sound as if they resemble regular cookies nutritionally—but they really do. Besides the price, there is very little difference between the fructose-sweetened and sugar-free cookies and the regular cookies listed above. In some cases the sugar-free or fructose sweetened cookies actually have more calories, more carbohydrate, or more fat than regular cookies.

When it comes to cookies, my advice is to buy what you really like (even better if they are good-tasting, reduced-fat, cookies), keep the serving size small, have some with a meal, and don't forget to include them in your carbohydrate gram total for the meal.

Canned Fruit

Even living in California, we find ourselves resorting to canned fruit to get us through the winter months. I always buy the no-sugar-added or "lite" fruit selections without hesitation. I didn't realize, until doing research for this chapter, just how many grams of carbohydrate you save by doing this—about 10 grams of carbohydrate and 30 to 40 calories per 1/2 cup serving. Here are some of the no-sugar-added canned fruit options available in many supermarkets. Considering that the fruit was canned, it tasted great to the taste testers.

Libby's Lite Pear Halves No Sugar Added (heavy syrup type contains 23 grams of carbohydrate and 90 calories)

Serving	Calories	Fat (g)	Saturated Fat (g)	Total Carbohydrate (g)	Fiber (g)
1/2 cup	60	0	0	13	1

Libby's Lite Sliced Peaches (heavy syrup type contains 24 grams of carbohydrate and 100 calories)

Serving	Calories	Fat (g)	Saturated Fat (g)	Total Carbohydrate (g)	Fiber (g)
¹/₂ cup	60	0	0	13	1

DelMonte Lite Apricot Halves with Extra Light Syrup (heavy syrup contains 27 grams of carbohydrate and 110 calories)

Serving	Calories	Fat (g)	Saturated Fat (g)	Total Carbohydrate (g)	Fiber (g)
¹/₂ cup	60	0	0	16	1

Dole Pineapple Chunks No Sugar Added (heavy syrup type contains 24 grams of carbohydrate and 90 calories)

Serving	Calories	Fat (g)	Saturated Fat (g)	Total Carbohydrate (g)	Fiber (g)
¹/₂ cup	60	0	0	15	1

Ice Cream

Edy's/Dreyer's, bless their heart, has tried to make no-sugar ice creams that are also fat-free. I say "tried to make" because after tasting these products—this taste wasn't ice cream to me. It tastes like something else, and I'm not sure what. The fat-free, no-sugar-added ice creams tend to have about 90 calories and 19 grams of carbohydrate for each ¹/₂-cup serving, whereas the reduced-fat, no-sugar-added ice creams contain about 100 calories and 16 grams of carbohydrate. So there really isn't any benefit to buying the yucky-tasting, fat-free, no-sugar ice creams. Do yourself a favor, buy the reduced-fat, no-sugar-added ice creams and enjoy yourself, knowing the extra 3 grams of fat per serving is well worth it for flavor. And you're actually saving yourself about 3 grams of carbohydrate per ¹/₂-cup serving!

Edy's/Dreyer's No Sugar Added Vanilla Ice Cream

Serving	Calories	Fat (g)	Saturated Fat (g)	Total Carbohydrate (g)	Sugar (g)
¹/₂ cup	100	3	1.5	15	4

Most tasters thought this vanilla was pretty good. There was a noticeable difference in flavor, but it was slight. While I prefer the taste of the light vanilla ice creams I've tasted, this one would do fine in a pinch.

Edy's/Dreyer's No Sugar Added Strawberry Ice Cream

Serving	Calories	Fat (g)	Saturated Fat (g)	Total Carbohydrate* (g)	Sugar (g)
½ cup	100	3	1.5	15	5

*Contains NutraSweet and sorbitol.

This tasted pretty good to most of the testers. I like that it contains real strawberries and real cream (although it is the sixth ingredient listed).

Edy's/Dreyer's No Sugar Added Triple Chocolate

Serving	Calories	Fat (g)	Saturated Fat (g)	Total Carbohydrate* (g)	Sugar (g)
½ cup	100	3	1.5	16	3

*Contains NutraSweet, maltitol, mannitol, and sorbitol.

This tasted pretty good to most of the testers. It probably won't have quite the intense chocolate flavor you were expecting in an ice cream called "triple chocolate," but it tasted fine for a plain old chocolate ice cream.

Ice Cream Bars

Eskimo Pie Reduced Fat, Sweetened with NutraSweet

Serving	Calories	Fat (g)	Saturated Fat (g)	Total Carbohydrate (g)	Sugar (g)
1 bar	120	8	6	13	3?

This tastes terrific, and it contains only 13 grams of carbohydrate. That's the good news. You know I'm warming you up for the bad news, don't you? It's bad enough that the grams of fat per bar are 8, which means the percent calories from fat for this minor indiscretion is 60 percent. But the second item in the ingredient list is coconut oil, a notoriously high saturated-fat oil—which explains why 6 of the 8 grams of fat are saturated (as shown above). In addition to NutraSweet, this product contains sorbitol and mannitol. If you can spare the 8 grams of fat, then this ice cream bar is a great-tasting treat.

Fudgsicles Sugar-Free (Good Humor) with NutraSweet

Serving	Calories	Fat (g)	Saturated Fat (g)	Total Carbohydrate (g)	Sugar (g)
1 bar	40	5	0	8	0

This tasted all right to most of the testers. The product tasted more like a chocolate ice-milk pop rather than a "fudge"-sicle, however. But that probably has more to do with this popsicle being very low in fat than it being sugar-free. Some of the testers said they might buy these again while others said they wouldn't.

Klondike Reduced Fat No Sugar Added with NutraSweet

Serving	Calories	Fat (g)	Saturated Fat (g)	Total Carbohydrate (g)	Sugar (g)
1 bar	190	10	7	19	?

These bars taste terrific! Everyone who tasted them loved them. In fact, you can't really notice a difference between these bars and the regular Klondike bars. Maybe that's because they still have 10 grams of fat. Makes you wonder—if the reduced-fat Klondike bars contain 10 grams of fat, how much fat is in the regular Klondike bars?

If you can spare the 190 calories and 10 grams of fat, these ice cream bars are a slice of heaven. If that's a bit much for you and your eating plan, try cutting them in half. You may find 95 calories and 5 grams of fat more feasible.

Nestlé Reduced Fat No Sugar Added Crunch Bars

Serving	Calories	Fat (g)	Saturated Fat (g)	Total Carbohydrate (g)	Sugar (g)
1 bar (50 g)	130	7	5	14	6

Some would say, gee, no sugar and reduced fat, what's the point! But these bars are pretty good tasting. You'll notice there are still 6 grams of sugar per bar. How could that be when there is no sugar added? The lactose, or milk sugar, in the skim milk (which is the second ingredient) contributes this amount. Sorbitol and NutraSweet are the sweeteners used. If you are wondering why the saturated fat is so high in this product, you have only to look at the first ingredient for the coating—coconut oil (one of the few naturally saturated oils).

No Sugar Added Pies

Marie Calender's No Sugar Added Pies*

Serving	Calories	Fat (g)	Saturated Fat (g)	Total Carbohydrate (g)
Lite Apple, 1/5 pie	722	50	N/A	54
Lite Strawberry, 1/4 pie	495	28	N/A	53
Razzleberry Lite, 1/5 pie	705	48	N/A	52
Peach Lite, 1/4 pie	481	27	N/A	55

*National restaurant chain

I tried these pies a bit skeptically after I choked down the Sara Lee No Sugar Added Cherry Pie—and once bitten, twice shy. They tasted almost the same as a regular sugar-sweetened pie. There was a slight artificial sweetener flavor with the strawberry pie and the apple pie. But many people probably wouldn't even notice the difference.

The peach and the strawberry lite pies have noticeably fewer calories than the others because they are one-crust pies. That top crust really loads on the extra calories and grams of fat. In fact, all these pies are just as high in fat as regular pies—so only the one-crust pies are going to save fat and calories.

All the pies have about the same amount of total carbohydrates per serving—from the fruit and flour.

Sara Lee Reduced Fat No Sugar Added Cherry (also Apple) Pie

Serving	Calories	Fat (g)	Saturated Fat (g)	Total Carbohydrate* (g)	Sugar (g)
¹⁄₆ pie (123 g)	220	8	1.5	35	5

*Contains NutraSweet

This tasted pretty good at first, and then the strong artificial sweetener taste invades your mouth. I ended up throwing the pie away. I'm not sure what Marie Calender's is doing differently, but their no-sugar-added pies taste great, with little noticeable aftertaste. Maybe Sara Lee needs to take cooking lessons from Marie Calender's.

Less Sugar Added

A handful of food products add less sugar than the original product. These products might boast a "lite" or "light" label, or a "less sugar" or "reduced sugar" name on the package. And in the case of Estee's peanut butter cups, chocolate bars, and other confections, the term "fructose sweetened" is used. In this case, though, they aren't technically adding less sugar; they are adding fructose instead, a sweetener that still contributes carbohydrate.

Hershey's Lite Chocolate Syrup (50% Fewer Calories and Sugar)

Serving	Calories	Total Carbohydrate (g)
2 Tb.	50	12

I tried to like this product; I really did. I liked the concept—a chocolate syrup that I could use in milk and on ice cream that had half as many calories and maybe half as much carbohydrate as regular chocolate syrup (like the light pancake syrups, which basically add water to regular pancake syrups).

But this product had a funny flavor to it ("funny" as in "strange"). The list of ingredients contained first water, then sugar, fructose, and cocoa (sounded all right so far). Then toward the bottom there was "a nonnutritive sweetener." Aha! That must be where the strange flavor came from. Either way, all of my tasters said they wouldn't buy this again. They would rather use half as much of the regular Hershey's chocolate syrup, which, by the way, contains 100 calories and 24 grams of carbohydrate per 2 tablespoon serving.

Jams

	Serving	Calories	Total Carbohydrate (g)
Smucker's Low Sugar	1 Tb.	25	6
(comes in grape, apricot, strawberry, and sweet orange)			
Smucker's Light Fruit Spread	1 Tb.	10	5
(contains NutraSweet, and comes in boysenberry, apricot, strawberry, and red raspberry)			
Smucker's Simply Fruit	1 Tb.	40	10
(assorted flavors)			
Knott's Berry Farm 100% Fruit	1 Tb.	40	10
(comes in apple and cinnamon, boysenberry, apricot, strawberry, blackberry, and boysenberry)			
Sorrell Ridge 100% Fruit	1 Tb.	36	9
(assorted flavors)			

Let's put all of this into perspective, shall we? Regular jam contains 50 calories and 13 grams of carbohydrate per tablespoon. Some of the all-fruit or 100-percent fruit spreads contain almost as many calories (40) and grams of carbohydrate (10) as regular jam. The calories and grams of carbohydrate are just coming from the concentrated fruit instead of the added sugar.

Most people are perfectly happy with the less-sugar jams. You get pretty much the same fruit flavor with a little less sugar. Some people also like the light fruit spreads where you are getting the same fruit flavor with NutraSweet in place of sugar. The texture of both of these types of jams/spreads is a little different, but it may not bother you or your family. If you decide to use the 100-percent fruit spreads, just remember to include them in your carbohydrate totals, because a couple of tablespoons can add up to 20 grams of carbohydrate.

Light Pancake Syrups

Serving	Calories	Carbohydrate (g)	Sodium (g)
1/4 cup	100	26	160

Most of the light pancake syrups taste fine. They are really just regular syrup that has been diluted with water. So the syrup has the same flavor, just a little less intense. The S & W 70% Reduced Calorie Maple Flavor Syrup, however, is going to taste different. It contains sorbitol and saccharin. The product does, however, contribute 60 calories per serving instead of 100, and 13 grams of carbohydrate instead of 26. Many of the taste testers discovered, however, that they would rather have a little less of the light syrup than to have a lot of the artificially sweetened syrup.

Peanut Butter Cups

Serving	Calories	Fat (g)	Saturated Fat (g)	Total Carbohydrate (g)	Sugar (g)
Estee Fructose Sweetened, 5 candies (38 g)	200	12	7	19	13
compared to:					
Reese's Peanut Butter Cup (38 g)	184	12	9	18	N/A

Peanut butter cups are one of my favorite candies, so I wasn't sure I was going to like this fructose-sweetened look-alike. Most testers agreed they tasted "all right," but not really like the real McCoy. What's more, when you compare the fructose-sweetened to the exact same amount of the Reese's version, the fructose-sweetened has even more calories and basically the same amount of fat and carbohydrate grams.

Comstock More Fruit Light Cherry Pie Filling or Topping

Serving	Calories	Fat (g)	Fiber (g)	Total Carbohydrate (g)	Sugar (g)
⅓ cup	60	0	0	13	11

The regular cherry filling and topping contain 90 calories per serving, whereas this light product contains 60. There are no artificial sweeteners added—just less sugar. Most testers thought it tasted pretty good. They did, however, notice that it was missing some sugar. But this didn't bother most of the testers, including me.

THE WINNER'S CIRCLE OF LIGHT PRODUCTS

I know sometimes it seems that almost everyone is telling you to lose weight. So, naturally you are curious about any light, low-fat, or fat-free food that comes down the pike. You are willing to try any product that might help stack the weight cards in your favor. Right? I have two words to say to you—buyer beware!

Many of these fat-free products are bubbling over with sugar. In many product categories, such as cookies, cakes, brownies, snack bars, and so forth, when manufacturers take out the fat, they put in *more* sugar. In many cases sugar becomes the first ingredient. It's not that they're conspiring against people with diabetes, it's that sugar, and sugar-containing ingredients, make pretty good replacements for fat. They add flavor, moisture, and texture.

Many of these fat-free and low-fat products also taste terrible. I would hate for you to spend your valuable money on some of these new products only to throw them away in disgust. Or worse, I would hate for you to give up on eating lower-fat foods because you have had so many bad experiences.

In the hopes of sparing you from buying many of these bad-tasting products (and saving you a few hundred dollars), I put together a list of the very best products my family and five other families (including one family with diabetes) tasted for my book *Taste vs. Fat*. These truly belong in the Winner's Circle of light products.

#1   Louis Rich 50% Less Fat Turkey Bacon

Now I know there are bacon purists out there who would rather have the real thing less often than resort to bacon made from turkeys. But to many families, including my own, Louis Rich Turkey Bacon *is* bacon. If you cook the turkey bacon in a thick, nonstick frypan, over low heat, flipping the strips over frequently and being careful not to let them burn or cook too quickly, it will have a crispy, melt-in-your-mouth texture almost like the real thing. Many people swear by this bacon—including me.

Serving Size	Calories	Fat (g)	Saturated Fat (g)	Cholesterol (mg)	Sodium (mg)	Carbohydrate (g)
1 slice (14 g)	30	2.5	0.5	10	190	0

#2   Betty Crocker Sweet Rewards Low-Fat Family Brownie Mix

I've made my share of brownies from scratch, but there is just something about a brownie mix, conveniently sitting in the pantry, that is very appealing. If you have to stock your kitchen with a brownie mix, Betty Crocker's new Low-Fat Fudge Brownie Mix is definitely the ticket. I made all the low-fat and nonfat brownie mixes on the market and brought them to my Jazzercise class to sample. Almost everyone liked the Betty Crocker brownie the best.

It had the best flavor and a chewy brownie texture that most of us look for in a brownie. Incidentally, this was one of the brownie mixes with the lowest percentage of calories from sugar (the other one was SnackWell's Low Fat Fudge Brownie Mix).

Serving Size	Calories	Fat (g)	Saturated Fat (g)	Choles- terol (mg)	Carbo- hydrate (mg)	Sugar (g)
1/18 mix, prepared	130	2.5	0.5	0	27	18

#3   Reduced-Fat Cheeses You're Going to Love

I love cheese. It's that simple. So, trust me when I tell you there is a handful of really great-tasting lower-fat cheeses. What's their secret? They don't go *too* low in fat. They still have a respectable amount of fat for a cheese, and so they tend to taste as good as cheese. By the way, the following cheeses contain less than a gram of carbohydrate per 1-ounce serving.

Serving Size	Calories	Fat (g)	Saturated Fat (g)	Choles- terol (mg)	Sodium (mg)
Cracker Barrel Light Sharp Cheddar, 1 oz.	90	6.0	4.0	20	240
Kraft 1/3 Less Fat Sharp Cheddar, 1 oz.	90	6.0	4.0	20	240
Sonoma Dairies Garlic Jack 50% Less Fat, 1 oz.	70	4.0	2.5	15	180
Sonoma Lite Jack, 1 oz.	70	4.0	2.5	15	180
Jarlsberg Lite (in the deli section), 1 oz.	70	3.5	2.0	10	130
Sargento Light Swiss, 1 oz.	80	4.0	2.5	15	50

#4   Hillshire Farm Deli Select Honey Ham

This is one great-tasting ham. Most tasters preferred this brand of ham to all the others.

Serving Size	Calories	Fat (g)	Saturated Fat (g)	Choles- terol (mg)	Carbo- hydrate (mg)	Sodium (g)
3 slices (28 g)	30	0.8	0.3	12	2	300

#5 Gallo Light Italian Dry Salame and Hormel Turkey Pepperoni

Sometimes people actually like light products better than the original fatty version. It doesn't happen often, but when it does you feel like dancing in the street. One such product is Gallo Light Salame. Every taster not only thought it tasted great, they all liked it better than regular salami. (Real salami has many more fat globules visible to the naked eye.)

Most tasters also loved Hormel's new 70 percent less fat Turkey Pepperoni, which definitely has a pepperonilike flavor but without all the grease.

Serving Size	Calories	Fat (g)	Saturated Fat (g)	Choles-terol (mg)	Carbo-hydrate (mg)	Sodium (g)
5 slices Gallo Light Salame (29 g, 1.02 oz.)	60	4.0		25	1	520
17 slices Hormel Turkey Pepperoni (30 g, 1.06 oz.)	80	4.0	1.5	40	0	550

#6 SnackWell's and Chips Ahoy Reduced Fat Chocolate Chip Cookies

It's important to know that you can buy a couple of good-tasting reduced-fat chocolate chip cookies, just in case you have a lunchbox to fill or you turn into the Cookie Monster from time to time. The Reduced Fat Chips Ahoy is a little lower in percentage of calories from sugar compared to the SnackWell's.

Serving Size	Calories	Fat (g)	Saturated Fat (g)	Carbo-hydrate (mg)
SnackWell's Reduced Fat Mini Chocolate Chip Cookies, 13 (29 g)	130	3.5	1.5	22
Reduced Fat Chips Ahoy, 3 (32 g)	140	6	1.5	22

#7 The Best-Tasting Creme Sandwich Cookies

SnackWell's makes it into the Winner's Circle yet again with its Reduced Fat Creme Sandwich Cookie. Elfin Delights 50% Reduced Fat Vanilla Cookies also taste great. Compared to other reduced-fat or fat-free cookies, they really aren't that high in sugar, either.

Serving Size	Calories	Fat (g)	Saturated Fat (g)	Carbo-hydrate (mg)
Elfin Delights 50% Reduced Fat Vanilla, 2 (25 g)	110	2.5	0.5	21
SnackWell's Reduced Fat Creme Sandwich Cookie, 2 (26 g)	110	2.5	0.5	21

#8   The Best-Tasting Cookie Dough

The best tasting reduced-fat chocolate chip cookie dough is, at this time, the only reduced-fat chocolate chip cookie dough. But it happens to taste darn good. It's SnackWell's Chocolate Chip Cookie Dough. Most every tester (even the pickier ones) really liked these cookies.

Serving Size	Calories	Fat (g)	Saturated Fat (g)	Carbo-hydrate (mg)	Choles-terol (mg)
1 oz.	110	3.0	1.5	19	<5

#9   The Best-Tasting Crackers

Reduced Fat Cheese Nips get my vote as the best-tasting cheese cracker, but some tasters also liked SnackWell's Reduced Fat Zesty Cheese crackers the best. Between the two, you are sure to find one you like.

Serving	Calories	Fat (g)	Saturated Fat (g)	Choles-terol (mg)	Carbo-hydrate (g)	Sodium (mg)
Reduced Fat Cheese Nips, 31 crackers (30 g)	130	3.5	1.0	0	21	310
SnackWell's Reduced Fat Zesty Cheese, 32 crackers (30 g)	120	2.0	0.5	<5	23	350

Everything tastes better sitting on a Ritz? Well, the reduced-fat Ritz will do, but according to our tasters, Keebler's Reduced Fat Club Crackers or Reduced Fat Hi-Ho Crackers may do a little better. Most people thought these two crackers showed little difference compared to the original high-fat crackers. You might have some trouble finding the reduced-fat Hi-Ho crackers though; I did.

Serving	Calories	Fat (g)	Saturated Fat (g)	Choles- terol (mg)	Carbo- hydrate (g)	Sodium (mg)
Keebler Reduced Fat Club crackers, 10 (32g)	140	4.0	0	0	24	400
Reduced Fat Hi-Ho, 10 (30 g)	140	5.0	1.0	0	22	280
Reduced Fat Ritz, 10 (30 g)	140	4.0	0	0	22	280

#10 The Best-Tasting Wheat Cracker—SnackWell's Does It Again

A tiscuit, a tasket, SnackWell's Fat Free Wheat Crackers in my basket. I was skeptical, I admit. Fat-free wheat crackers? But somehow, SnackWell's managed to create a nice-tasting, flaky wheat cracker that stole the hearts of many of my tasters.

Serving	Calories	Fat (g)	Saturated Fat (g)	Choles- terol (mg)	Carbo- hydrate (g)	Sodium (mg)
SnackWell's Fat Free Wheat Crackers, 10 (30 g)	120	0	0	0	24	340

#11 Reduced Fat Crescent Roll Dough

Lately I've been appreciating the merits of a package of ready-to-go crescent roll dough in my refrigerator. I can make dinner rolls or pigs in a blanket (using light hot dogs, of course) in a moment's notice. But regular crescent roll dough is loaded with fat. Well, now you have a couple of options. You can choose Pillsbury Reduced Fat Crescent Roll dough or you can opt for the store brand for a crescent roll dough that is often even lower in fat than the Pillsbury reduced-fat version. In addition to our six families, I also tested both types on a classroom of five-year-olds and a handful of adults. Everyone liked them.

Serving	Calories	Fat (g)	Saturated Fat (g)	Choles- terol (mg)	Carbo- hydrate (g)	Sodium (mg)
Pillsbury Reduced Fat Crescent Rolls 1 roll	100	4.5	1.0	0	12	230
store brand 1 roll	80	3.0	1.0	0	13	250

#12   Philadelphia Light Cream Cheese

If you are looking for a lower-fat cream cheese that is sure to please even the pickiest of palates, try Philadelphia Light Cream Cheese. It's great for everything from bagels to cheesecake.

Serving	Calories	Fat (g)	Saturated Fat (g)	Choles- terol (mg)	Carbo- hydrate (g)	Sodium (mg)
2 Tb.	70	5.0	3.5	15	2	150

#13   The Best-Tasting Egg Substitute—Egg Beaters

In the case of egg substitutes, newer isn't necessarily better. One of the oldest egg substitutes on the market, Egg Beaters, is still the best-tasting egg substitute. Egg Beaters is made from mostly egg white with vegetable gums added for thickening and beta carotene for color. It looks and tastes more like real eggs than the other substitutes. I like to use half Egg Beaters and half real eggs when making scrambled eggs, omelets, or quiche. This cuts the fat and cholesterol in half, with only a slight difference in taste and texture.

Serving	Calories	Fat (g)	Saturated Fat (g)	Choles- terol (mg)	Carbo- hydrate (g)	Sodium (mg)
1/4 cup	30	0	0	0	1	100

#14   The Best-Tasting Frozen Entrees

It took just about every ounce of open-mindedness I could muster to remain part of the test group and taste the frozen entrée selections. I know many people live on this stuff—but I don't. The thought of frozen prepared food that contains anywhere from twenty-five to sixty ingredients and additives just doesn't appeal to me, since I make it a habit to cook dinner from scratch. However, I found a couple of frozen entrées that tasted pretty good, even to me. These select few are listed below.

Serving	Calories	Fat (g)	Saturated Fat (g)	Choles- terol (mg)	Carbo- hydrate (g)	Sodium (mg)
Healthy Choice Chicken Fettuccine Alfredo, 1	260	4.5	2.0	40	35	410
Lean Cuisine Chicken Fettuccine, 1	270	6.0	2.5	45	38	580

Serving	Calories	Fat (g)	Saturated Fat (g)	Choles- terol (mg)	Carbo- hydrate (g)	Sodium (mg)
Lean Cuisine Chicken Piccata, 1	290	6.0	1.5	30	45	540
Healthy Choice Garlic Chicken Milano, 1	240	4.0	2.0	35	34	510

#15 The Best-Tasting Less-Fat Franks (Hot Dogs)

My family has two brands of lower-fat franks that we buy regularly. They even pass muster with the man of the house. The testers agreed these two were the best tasting. Most tasters thought they would buy either one of these again. That's high praise for a leaner wiener!

Serving	Calories	Fat (g)	Saturated Fat (g)	Choles- terol (mg)	Carbo- hydrate (g)	Sodium (mg)
Ball Park Lite, 1	110	8.0	2.0	20	4	730
Louis Rich Turkey Franks, 1	110	8.0	2.5	50	2	630

#16 The Best-Tasting Light Ice Creams

Certain light ice creams were a big hit with almost every taster. Here they are.

Serving (1/2 cup)	Calories	Fat (g)	Saturated Fat (g)	Choles- terol (mg)	Carbo- hydrate (g)
Breyer's Light Vanilla	130	4.5	3.0	35	18
Edy's/Dreyer's Grand Light Rocky Road	110	4.0	2.0	20	16
Dreyer's Grand Light Expresso Fudge Chip	110	4.0	2.5	15	18
Healthy Choice Special Creations Cappuccino Mocha Fudge	120	2.0	1.0	<5	23
Healthy Choice Special Creations Cherry Chocolate Chunk	110	2.0	1.0	<5	N/A
Healthy Choice Special Creations Turtle Fudge Cake	130	2.0	1.0	<5	25
Ben & Jerry's Low Fat Cherry Garcia	170	3.0	2.0	10	31

#17   The Best-Tasting Diet Margarine—I Can't Believe It's Not Butter

Diet margarine comes in handy for spreading on toast, muffins, biscuits, waffles, potatoes, and for even making homemade frosting. In other cases it doesn't work as well as stick butter or margarine because of its high water content. But if you are going to try a diet margarine, why not try the best-tasting one?

Serving	Calories	Fat (g)	Saturated Fat (g)	Choles-terol (mg)	Sodium (mg)
1 Tb.	50	6.0	1.0	0	90

#18   Best Foods/Hellmann's Light and Low-Fat Mayonnaise

Some people just don't like the lower-fat mayonnaises. If you are one of those, try to use much less of the real thing. You can use a blend of real mayonnaise with your favorite fat-free sour cream for potato, macaroni, or shrimp salads. Otherwise, give Best Foods/Hellmann's Light or Low Fat mayonnaise a go. These were the top two reduced-fat mayonnaises with our tasters.

Serving	Calories	Fat (g)	Saturated Fat (g)	Choles-terol (mg)	Carbo-hydrate (g)	Sodium (mg)
Best Foods/Hellmann's Light, 1 Tb.	50	5.0	1.0	5	1	115
Best Foods/Hellmann's Low Fat, 1 Tb.	25	1.0	0	0	4	140

#19   Reduced-Fat JIF Peanut Butter

Using a little peanut butter on toast is a good way for people with diabetes to help add a little protein and fat to a normally high-carbohydrate breakfast. Reduced-Fat JIF was considered the best-tasting reduced-fat peanut butter by almost every taster. Some tasters even liked it better than regular JIF.

Serving	Calories	Fat (g)	Saturated Fat (g)	Choles-terol (mg)	Carbo-hydrate (g)	Sodium (mg)
2 Tb.	190	12	2.5	0	15	250

#20   When You've Got to Have a Potato Chip—Reach for These

As long as you aren't too terribly picky about potato chips, you should be quite happy with Reduced Fat Lay's or Pringles Right Crisps when you've just got to have one (or two). These two lower-fat chips are by no means "low in fat," but they do have a few grams less fat per ounce.

Serving	Calories	Fat (g)	Saturated Fat (g)	Choles-terol (mg)	Carbo-hydrate (g)	Sodium (mg)
Reduced Fat Lay's, 1 oz.	140	6.7	1.0	0	19	130
Pringles Right Crisps, 1 oz.	140	7.0	2.0	0	19	135

#21   Precious Low-Fat Ricotta Cheese

For those times when you're making lasagna, manicotti, or ravioli, reach for the Precious low-fat ricotta cheese and save yourself a bit of fat and calories without forsaking taste and texture.

Serving	Calories	Fat (g)	Saturated Fat (g)	Choles-terol (mg)	Carbo-hydrate (g)	Sodium (mg)
1/4 cup	70	3.0	1.5	15	3	45

#22   Hidden Valley Ranch Light Original Ranch and Three Great Light Vinaigrettes

It's difficult finding a great-tasting bottled salad dressing. But let's face it, some of us don't find the time to make salad dressings from scratch, unless it's a special occasion. I did find one light creamy dressing and three light vinaigrette dressings that most every taster liked—Hidden Valley Ranch Light Original Ranch and Wish-Bone Olive Oil Vinaigrette, Lawrys Classic Red Wine Vinaigrette, and Seven Seas Reduced Fat Red Wine Vinegar & Oil.

If your favorite dressing is something like Cardini's or Girard's Caesar dressing with 16 grams of fat per 2 tablespoons, try blending it with the same amount of lowfat milk for a thinner, tasty dressing with half the fat. Most salad dressings contain between 2 and 4 grams of carbohydrate per 2-tablespoon serving.

Serving	Calories	Fat (g)	Saturated Fat (g)	Choles- terol (mg)	Sodium (mg)
Hidden Valley Ranch Light Original Ranch, 2 Tb.	80	7	0.5	0	270
Wish-Bone Olive Oil Vinaigrette, 2 Tb.	60	5	1.0	0	250
Lawrys Classic Red Wine Vinaigrette, 2 Tb.	90	7	1.0	0	480
Seven Seas Reduced Fat Red Wine Vinegar & Oil, 2 Tb.	45	4	0.5	0	320

Make a Quick & Tasty Ranch Dressing

In a bowl, mix 1 packet Hidden Valley Ranch Salad Dressing Mix (1 oz.) with 1 cup low-fat milk, $^1/_2$ cup mayonnaise, and $^1/_2$ cup fat-free sour cream (or use 1 cup light mayo and fat-free sour cream). Mix well. Cover and refrigerate at least 30 minutes. Stir before serving. Makes 2 cups dressing that stays fresh 3 to 4 weeks.

	Calories	Fat (g)	Saturated Fat (g)	Cholesterol (mg)	Sodium (mg)
2 Tb.	68	5.5	0.8	3.5	197

#23   Jimmy Dean Light Sausage and Jones Light Pork and Rice Links

If you want a sausage that looks and tastes like real sausage but has a little less fat (one-third to one-half less), then Jimmy Dean Light and Jones Light Pork and Rice Links just may become your new favorite sausages. Some tasters even liked the Jones Light Pork and Rice Links better than real sausage links because they didn't have as much grease.

Serving	Calories	Fat (g)	Saturated Fat (g)	Choles- terol (mg)	Sodium (mg)
Jimmy Dean Light, uncooked (75 g)	180	14.0	1.0	55	500
Jones Light Pork and Rice Links, 2 links (56 g)	130	11.0	4.0	20	420

#24 Hillshire Farm Lite Smoked Sausage (Large Link)

Most every taster preferred this sausage to the other lower-fat large link sausages.

Serving	Calories	Fat (g)	Saturated Fat (g)	Choles- terol (mg)	Sodium (mg)
2 oz.	120	8.0	4.5	25	510

#25 Soup—Healthy Choice New England Clam Chowder

Most every taster liked this lower-fat clam chowder the best. It has a nice, peppery flavor and an appetizing texture to it.

Serving	Calories	Fat (g)	Saturated Fat (g)	Choles- terol (mg)	Carbo- hydrate (g)	Sodium (mg)
1 cup ready-to-eat	120	1.5	1.0	10	23	480

#26 Naturally Yours Fat-Free Sour Cream (available on West Coast)

I know it sounds too good to be true—a nonfat sour cream with a nice taste and texture. But that's exactly what I found in Naturally Yours Fat-Free Sour Cream. It even tasted better than some of the light sour creams. Use it in casseroles, for dips, in soups, or anywhere your spoon takes you. (It's the one in the black-and-white cowhide container.)

Serving	Calories	Fat (g)	Saturated Fat (g)	Choles- terol (mg)	Sodium (mg)
2 Tb.	20	0	0	0	50

The following is a bonus addition to the Winner's Circle of Light Products, nominated by my group of taste testers with diabetes. I include it, or rather them, because pasta is such an important part of a diabetes meal plan.

27 The Best-Tasting Bottled Spaghetti Sauces

While buying my favorite bottled spaghetti sauce at my local supermarket yesterday, I was reminded just how liberating good-tasting spaghetti sauce in a bottle really is. The checker with an Italian-sounding last name looked at my choice of spaghetti sauce and commented, "Isn't this a great sauce; I don't have to make my sauce from scratch anymore." That made me think, you know, there really are some great-tasting bottled spaghetti sauces now. And what a relief it is to be able to reach into the refrigerator or pantry when a little red sauce is needed for a quick batch of spaghetti, ravioli, or homemade pizza.

My personal favorite is Classico di Napoli Roasted Garlic. Now, I know spaghetti sauce is a very personal thing. Some of us like our sauce loaded with chunks of onion. Some of us like a splash of wine or a sweet/sour flavor in our sauce. Some of us like the mature taste of sauce that has been simmering for hours, while others prefer the fresh, just-cooked type of sauce. Listed below are the four spaghetti sauce selections rated as excellent by my taste testers. No matter what your sauce preference—these selections should give you a nice range of sauces to choose from.

Serving (1/2 cup)	Calories	Fat (g)	Sodium (mg)	Carbo-hydrate (g)	Fiber (g)
Safeway Select Mushroom & Onion	60	3.0	510	6	1
Classico di Napoli Tomato & Basil	50	1.0	410	8	2
Classico di Napoli Roasted Garlic	60	1.5	390	9	2
Newman's Own Bombolina (great fresh basil flavor)	100	4.0	590	15	5

8

RECIPES YOU NEED AND RECIPES YOU ASKED FOR

I asked members of diabetic support groups what meals they like to eat and what foods they missed the most. Not surprisingly, I received many requests for desserts and a few tasty and presumed forbidden favorites like Chinese chicken salad. That's why the recipes I've provided here include a hefty selection of sweet things, although the recipes themselves are both light and satisfying.

I also wanted to offer a variety of recipes that would meet the experts' recommendations for healthy meal plans. You'll find recipes high in soluble fiber featuring oat bran (bread, pancakes, even pizza) or beans (some Mexican classics). Pasta recipes are here because they have low glycemic indexes compared to other carbohydrate-rich entrées. Cholesterol-lowering mono-unsaturated fat is represented in several Mediterranean dishes and salads.

All the recipes have been taste-tested and judged worthy. You may not like every one, but you should enjoy most. For each recipe, I've listed the relevant nutritional data: number of calories and calories from fat; grams of carbohydrate, fat, fiber, and protein; and milligrams of cholesterol and sodium. This information should be very valuable in designing and following your meal plan.

Enjoy!

Recipes to Wake Up To	Page
Mexican Quiche	179
Deluxe Granola	180
Traditional Two Eggs and Hash Brown Breakfast	180
Cinnamon Rolls	181
Almond Oat Bran Muffins	182

Recipes to Wake Up To	Page
Quick Ham and Cheese Turnovers	183
Banana Bread	183
Light Oat Bran Pancakes	184
Reduced-Fat Bisquick Waffles	185
Reduced-Fat Bisquick Buttermilk Pancakes	185
Hot Maple Oat Bran Cereal	186

Side Dishes

Oat Bran Corn Bread	187
Grandma's Traditional Bread Stuffing	187
Roasted Vegetables	188
Ozark Pumpkin Bread	189
Garden Sauté	189
High Mono Green Salad	190
Spinach and Blue Cheese Salad (with toasted almonds)	190
Saffron Rice	191

Snacks

Seven-Layer Mexican Dip	191
Easy Roasted Potatoes	192
Quick French Onion Dip	193

Entrées

Oat Bran Pizza	193
Oat Bran Bread	194
Antipasto Sandwich	195
Quick and Crustless Vegetable Quiche	195
Chicken Prosciutto	196
Chicken and Cabbage Ramen Salad	197
Mexican Pizza	198
Super Quick Pesto Pasta	199
Soluble Fiber Meat Loaf	199
Beef Tacos	200
Simple Salmon Pasta Salad	201
Chinese Chicken Salad	201
Salad Niçoise	202
Salmon Burgers	203
Ranch Vegetable Chicken Salad	204
Quick-Fix Schilling Chili	204
Chicken-Mango-Avocado Salad	205

Desserts

Light Chocolate Cake   205
Frozen Light Lemon Pie   207
Apple-Oat Crisp   207
Choc-Oat-Chip Bars   208
Very Berry Ice Cream   209
Strawberry Shortcake   209
Cocoa Brownies   210
Soft Chocolate Chip Cookies   211
Blender Chocolate Mousse   211
Apricot Dessert Bars   212
Peanut Butter Oat Bran Bars   213

RECIPES TO WAKE UP TO

Mexican Quiche

Makes 8 servings.
Nonstick cooking spray
5 eggs
$1/2$ cup flour
1 teaspoon baking powder
Dash salt
$1^1/4$ cup fat-free egg substitute
$1/2$ cup low-fat milk
2 cans (4 ounces) chopped green chiles (mild, medium, or hot)
2 cups low-fat cottage cheese, whipped in food processor until smooth
12 ounces reduced-fat jack cheese, grated
salsa

Preheat oven to 400°. Coat a large casserole (or 9-by-13-inch baking pan) with nonstick cooking spray; set aside.

In mixer bowl, combine the eggs, flour, baking powder, and salt, and beat well. Add egg substitute and milk, and beat until smooth. Stir in green chiles, cottage cheese, and grated cheese. Pour into prepared pan and bake for 15 minutes, then reduce heat to 350° and bake for 30 minutes more. Serve with salsa.

Per serving: 259 calories, 12 g carbohydrates, 11 g fat, 1 g fiber, 27 g protein, 161 mg cholesterol, 610 mg sodium. *Calories from fat:* 38%.

Deluxe Granola

Makes 13 half-cup servings.

3 tablespoons canola oil
$^1/_3$ cup honey
1 cup apple juice
1 teaspoon vanilla
$^1/_2$ teaspoon cinnamon
4 cups old-fashioned oats
$^1/_3$ cup raw slivered almonds or pecans
$^1/_2$ cup roasted sunflower seeds
$^1/_2$ cup roasted cashew pieces
$^2/_3$ cup raisins
$^1/_2$ cup flaked or shredded coconut

Directions Using Oven

Preheat oven to 350°. In small saucepan over medium-low heat, cook 2 tablespoons oil with honey, apple juice, vanilla, and cinnamon until well blended.

Line a jelly roll pan with foil and spread remaining tablespoon of oil evenly over it. Add oats and almonds or pecans to pan.

Drizzle honey mixture over the top of oats in pan. Stir to blend. Bake or cook for 20 minutes, stirring twice. Add oat mixture to mixing bowl. Stir in remaining ingredients.

Directions Using Electric Skillet

Preheat skillet to 340°. Add 3 tablespoons oil to skillet and spread to coat. Stir in honey, then slowly stir in apple juice, vanilla, and cinnamon. Continue to stir until well blended. Stir in oats and almonds or pecans. Let cook, stirring frequently until oats and nuts lightly brown (15 to 20 minutes). Turn off the heat and stir in remaining ingredients. Once cool, completely store in Ziploc bags.

Per serving: 247 calories, 32 g carbohydrates, 11 g fat, 4 g fiber, 7 g protein, 0 mg cholesterol, about 100 mg sodium (depending on the nuts you use). *Calories from fat: 39%.*

Traditional Two Eggs and Hash Brown Breakfast

Makes 1 serving.

$1^1/_2$ teaspoons canola oil
2 cups Oreida Country Style hash browns

Nonstick cooking spray
Herbs to taste, such as Italian seasoning or other herb blends, or parsley
  (optional)
$^1/_2$ cup Egg Beaters egg substitute
Pepper to taste
Fresh chopped or sliced tomato (optional)

Heat oil in nonstick skillet or frypan over medium heat. Spread oil
with spatula to cover pan evenly. Add frozen hash browns to form an
even layer. Spray top of hash browns with nonstick cooking spray. Fry
5 minutes, then turn hash browns over to fry 2 minutes longer. Season
top of hash browns with fresh or dried herbs, if desired. Transfer hash
browns from frypan to plate.

Spray same pan with nonstick cooking spray. Add egg substitute
and scramble, or let cook like an omelette. Add pepper or parsley to
taste. Serve hash browns with eggs and fresh tomato, if desired.

Per serving: 240 calories, 30 g carbohydrate, 7 g fat, 2 g fiber, 16 g
protein, 0 mg cholesterol, 240 mg sodium. *Calories from fat: 26%.*

Cinnamon Rolls

Makes 12 rolls.

1 box (16 oz) Pillsbury Hot Roll Mix (includes yeast packet)
3 packets Sweet 'n Low
3 tablespoons sugar
1 egg
1 tablespoon canola oil
1 cup hot water, 120 to 130 degrees (very hot to touch)
$^1/_3$ cup pecan or walnut pieces
2 teaspoons cinnamon
3 tablespoon diet margarine (such as I Can't Believe It's Not Butter Light)
1 tablespoon corn syrup or honey
$^1/_2$ teaspoon vanilla
Nonstick cooking spray

Glaze
$^1/_2$ cup powdered sugar
2 to 4 teaspoons low-fat milk
$^1/_4$ teaspoon vanilla

Combine hot roll mix, yeast packet, 1 packet Sweet 'n Low, and 1
tablespoon sugar in a large bowl; mix well. Stir in hot water, egg, and
canola oil until dough pulls away from sides of bowl. Turn dough out

onto lightly floured surface. With floured hands, shape dough into a
ball. Knead dough for 5 minutes until smooth. Cover dough with large
bowl; let rest 5 minutes.

Meanwhile, in small food processor or blender, grind pecans, 2
packets Sweet 'n Low, 2 tablespoons sugar, and cinnamon briefly until
blended; set aside. Blend diet margarine with corn syrup and vanilla;
set aside.

Coat a 13-by-9-inch pan with nonstick cooking spray. To shape
dough, roll it to about a 15-by-10-inch rectangle. Spread the margarine mixture evenly over the dough. Sprinkle with pecan-cinnamon
mixture. Start with 10-inch side and roll up tightly, pressing edges to
seal. Cut with serrated knife into 12 slices; place, cut side down, in
prepared pan. Cover loosely with plastic wrap and cloth towel. Let
rise in warm place 30 minutes. Heat oven to 375°. Uncover rolls.
Bake for 20 minutes, or until golden brown.

To make glaze, combine powdered sugar, milk, and vanilla. Blend
until smooth and of drizzling consistency. Drizzle over warm rolls.

Per serving: 220 calories, 35.5 g carbohydrate, 6 g fat, 1 g fiber, 4.5 g
protein, 17 mg cholesterol, 270 mg sodium. *Calories from fat: 26%.*

Almond Oat Bran Muffins

Makes 12 muffins.

Nonstick cooking spray
2 cups oat bran
1 cup All-Bran cereal, processed briefly in food processor
1$\frac{1}{4}$ cups all-purpose flour
$\frac{1}{2}$ cup sugar
1$\frac{1}{2}$ teaspoons baking soda
$\frac{1}{4}$ teaspoon salt
1 egg
1 cup buttermilk
$\frac{1}{4}$ cup low-fat milk
3 tablespoons nonfat sour cream
3 tablespoons canola oil
1$\frac{1}{2}$ teaspoons almond extract

Preheat oven to 400°. Coat 12 muffin pan cups with nonstick cooking
spray and set them aside. In mixer bowl, blend first six ingredients. In
small bowl, beat egg, buttermilk, low-fat milk, sour cream, oil, and
almond extract with a fork until thoroughly blended.

Stir or beat egg mixture into flour mixture just until dry ingredients are moistened. Spoon batter into prepared muffin cups (about $1/4$ slightly heaping cup of batter per muffin cup). Bake 15 minutes, or until lightly browned. Immediately remove muffins from pan.

Per muffin: 187 calories, 36 g carbohydrate, 5.5 g fat, 5.5 g fiber, 6.7 g protein, 19 mg cholesterol, 315 mg sodium. *Calories from fat: 26%.*

Quick Ham and Cheese Turnovers

Makes 4 turnovers.

$1/2$ cup chopped thinly sliced lean ham
1 green onion, finely chopped
$1/3$ cup grated part-skim or reduced-fat Swiss or other cheese
$1/4$ cup fat-free egg substitute
1 pop can crescent dinner rolls (80 calories per 28-gram roll, and 3 g fat)

Preheat oven to 375°. Add first four ingredients to a medium-size bowl and toss to blend. Pop crescent roll can and unroll the dough. Separate the dough into 8 triangles. Place one of the triangles on a baking sheet. Top it with $1/8$ cup of the ham mixture. Lay another triangle over the first triangle so they match. Crimp the edges together with a cake fork.

Repeat with remaining dough and ham filling. Bake 10 to 15 minutes, or until golden brown.

Per turnover: 212 calories, 27 g carbohydrate, 7.5 g fat, 2 g fiber, 12 g protein, 12 mg cholesterol, 800 mg sodium. *Calories from fat: 32%.*

Banana Bread

Makes 10 slices.

This banana bread has 50 percent less sugar and is low in fat, compared to other banana bread recipes.

$1/3$ cup fat-free cream cheese
$1/2$ cup sugar
2 tablespoons canola oil
2 tablespoons dark rum or any juice
1 egg plus 1 egg white, or $1/8$ cup fat-free egg substitute
2 teaspoons vanilla
$13/4$ cups all-purpose flour
3 teaspoons baking powder

$^1/_2$ teaspoon salt
1 cup mashed very ripe bananas (about 3 medium)

Preheat oven to 350°. In large bowl of mixer, beat cream cheese for a minute until creamy. Gradually add sugar, beating until light and fluffy. Add the oil and rum or juice, and beat until smooth. Add egg, egg white, and vanilla; beat until thick (a few minutes).

In large mixing bowl, whisk together flour, baking powder, and salt. Slowly begin adding the flour mixture to the sugar mixture, alternating with the mashed bananas and combining well after each addition.

Coat a $4^1/_2$-by-$8^1/_2$-inch loaf pan with nonstick cooking spray. Pour the batter into the loaf pan and bake for about 45 minutes, or until cake tester comes out clean when inserted into the middle of the loaf. Cool 10 minutes before removing it from the pan. Cool completely on a wire rack.

This bread freezes and toasts well and is great with light cream cheese.

Per slice: 188 calories, 33 g carbohydrate, 3.5 g fat, 1 g fiber, 5 g protein, 22 mg cholesterol, 308 mg sodium. *Calories from fat:* 17%.

Light Oat Bran Pancakes

Makes 4 servings, 3 pancakes each.

These pancakes are high in fiber!
2 cups Krusteaz Lite Oat Bran Pancake Mix*
$^1/_2$ cup low-fat buttermilk
1 cup water
Canola nonstick cooking spray

Add pancake mix, buttermilk, and water to mixer bowl. Blend on medium-low mixer speed until just mixed. Heat heavy nonstick griddle or skillet over medium-low heat or preheat griddle to 375°. Coat frypan or griddle with canola nonstick cooking spray. Pour slightly less than $^1/_4$ cup of batter for each pancake. Cook pancakes about 1 minute per side or until golden brown, turning only once. These pancakes can be frozen in a Ziploc bag. Just heat in microwave on High for a minute or two to warm, or place in toaster.

*Krusteaz is available on the West Coast. Write company for ordering information: Continental Mills, Inc., P.O. Box 88176, Seattle, WA 93138-2176.

Per serving: 152 calories, 36 g carbohydrate, 1.3 g fat, 7 g fiber, 7 g protein, 1 mg cholesterol, 422 mg sodium. *Calories from fat: 8%.*

Reduced-Fat Bisquick Waffles

Makes 3 large waffles, or four 4-inch quarters.

2 cups Bisquick Reduced Fat baking mix
$1/3$ cup low-fat buttermilk or 1-percent or skim milk
1 cup 1-percent or skim milk
$1/4$ cup fat-free egg substitute
1 tablespoon canola oil
Canola nonstick cooking spray

Preheat waffle iron. Use a mixer to blend first five ingredients until smooth. Coat waffle iron with canola nonstick cooking spray. Pour batter onto hot waffle iron according to waffle iron directions. Bake until steaming stops.

Tip: Freeze leftover waffles in a Ziploc bag. To reheat, just place frozen waffles in toaster until crisp.

Per serving: 396 calories, 61 g carbohydrate, 10.5 g fat, 2 g fiber, 12 g protein, 4 mg cholesterol, 1,060 mg sodium. *Calories from fat: 24%.*

Reduced-Fat Bisquick Buttermilk Pancakes

Makes 4 servings, 3 pancakes each.

2 cups Bisquick Reduced Fat baking mix
$1/3$ cup low-fat buttermilk, or 1-percent skim milk
$3/4$ cup 1-percent or skim milk
$1/2$ cup fat-free egg substitute
Canola nonstick cooking spray

Use a mixer to blend first four ingredients until smooth. Begin heating a nonstick skillet or griddle over medium-low heat. Coat generously with canola nonstick cooking spray. Pour by $1/4$ cupfuls onto frypan or hot griddle. Cook until edges are dry. Turn; cook until golden.

For thinner pancakes, use $1/2$ cup buttermilk and 1 cup 1-percent or skim milk. For fluffier pancakes, add 2 tablespoons lemon juice, 4 teaspoons sugar, and 2 teaspoons baking powder.

Tip: Leftover pancakes can be frozen in Ziploc bags. To reheat, microwave frozen pancakes on High until hot or use a toaster.

Per serving: 269 calories, 45 g carbohydrate, 4.5 g fat, 2 g fiber, 10 g protein, 3 mg cholesterol, 850 mg sodium. *Calories from fat: 15%.*

Hot Maple Oat Bran Cereal

Makes 1 serving.

$^1/_2$ cup low-fat milk
$^1/_2$ cup water
$^1/_3$ cup 100% oat bran
$^1/_8$ teaspoon salt (optional)
pinch ground cinnamon (optional)
$^1/_2$ teaspoon vanilla extract
1 to 2 tablespoons light pancake syrup

Bring milk and water to a boil in a small saucepan. Stir in oat bran, salt, cinnamon, and vanilla, then cook for 1 to 2 minutes, stirring occasionally. Spoon cereal into bowl and drizzle syrup over the top.

Per serving (using 1 tablespoon of the light syrup): 205 calories, 42 g carbohydrate, 5.5 g fat, 7.3 g fiber, 12 g protein, 12 mg cholesterol, 110 mg sodium. *Calories from fat: 24%.*

SIDE DISHES

Oat Bran Corn Bread

Makes 9 servings.

Nonstick cooking spray
1 cup oat bran
1$^1/_2$ cups yellow cornmeal
1 cup all-purpose flour
1 teaspoon baking powder
1$^1/_2$ teaspoons baking soda
1 teaspoon salt
$^1/_4$ cup egg substitute
1$^3/_4$ cups low-fat buttermilk
5 tablespoons honey
3 tablespoons canola oil
$^1/_4$ cup fat-free or light sour cream

Preheat oven to 350°. Coat a 9-inch square pan with nonstick cooking spray.

In medium-size bowl, whisk together the oat bran, cornmeal, flour, baking powder, baking soda, and salt. In a mixing bowl, beat the egg substitute, buttermilk, honey, oil, and sour cream together. On low speed, slowly blend in dry ingredients, being careful not to overbeat. Pour into prepared pan. Bake for 30 minutes, or until the top of the corn bread is golden. Cut into squares and serve!

Per serving: 280 calories, 52 g carbohydrate, 6 g fat, 3 g fiber, 8 g protein, 2 mg cholesterol, 568 mg sodium. *Calories from fat: 18%.*

Grandma's Traditional Bread Stuffing

Makes 6 servings.

This is a variation on Grandma's traditional bread stuffing. Using oat bran bread increases the soluble fiber in this holiday favorite.

$^1/_2$ loaf oat bran or oatmeal bread (about 11 slices)
3 tablespoons butter or margarine
1 small onion, finely chopped
1 cup chopped celery
1 cup grated carrot
$^1/_8$ to $^1/_4$ teaspoon pepper

2 teaspoons poultry seasoning
1 tablespoon fresh chopped parsley
1 cup chicken broth

> Toast bread lightly. Cut into medium-size cubes. Melt butter in large skillet. Add onion, celery, carrot, pepper, and poultry seasoning. Simmer until celery is tender. Add parsley and mix in bread cubes. Drizzle $^1/_2$ cup chicken broth over the top and stir. If more chicken broth is desired for a moister stuffing, continue adding remaining broth, 2 tablespoons at a time. Cover pan and turn off heat. Let stuffing sit for 5 to 10 minutes to blend flavors.

> **Per serving:** 207 calories, 27 g carbohydrates, 8.3 g fat, 6 g fiber, 7 g protein, 15 mg cholesterol, 435 mg sodium. *Calories from fat:* 36%.

Roasted Vegetables

Makes 5 servings.

2 tablespoons olive oil
1 packet or cube regular or low-sodium chicken broth reconstituted with $^1/_4$ cup hot water
$^1/_2$ teaspoon fines herbes or other herb blend
$^1/_4$ teaspoon black pepper
1 tablespoon dried minced onions
2 to 3 cloves garlic, pressed or minced
3 medium-large potatoes, cut into bite-sized chunks, cooked on High in microwave for 10 minutes
4 carrots, cut into $^1/_2$-inch slices
About 1$^1/_2$ cups asparagus pieces or 2 cups julienne-cut zucchini

> Preheat oven to 400°. Coat bottom of 9-by-13-inch pan with 1 tablespoon of olive oil. Add remaining olive oil, chicken broth, herbs, pepper, onion, and garlic to 1- or 2-cup measure, and stir to blend well.

> Add potato pieces, carrot slices, and asparagus pieces to prepared baking pan. Drizzle chicken broth mixture over the top and toss vegetables well to mix and coat. Bake for 20 minutes, stirring after 10 minutes.

> **Per serving:** 223 calories, 39 g carbohydrate, 6 g fat, 5.5 g fiber, 5 g protein, 0 mg cholesterol, 250 mg sodium. *Calories from fat:* 24%.

Ozark Pumpkin Bread

Makes 9 servings.

The usual recipe contains 300 calories per serving, with 9 grams fat and 47 milligrams cholesterol.

Nonstick cooking spray
1 2/3 cups sifted flour
1/4 teaspoon baking powder
1 teaspoon baking soda
1/8 teaspoon salt
1 1/2 teaspoons pumpkin pie spice
3 tablespoons canola oil
3 tablespoons low-fat buttermilk
1 cup sugar
1 teaspoon vanilla
1 egg
1/4 cup egg substitute
1 cup canned pumpkin
1/3 cup sherry
Pecan halves (optional)

Preheat oven to 350°. Coat a 9-by-5-inch loaf pan with nonstick cooking spray. Blend flour, baking powder, baking soda, salt, and pumpkin pie spice together in medium-size bowl. In mixer bowl, cream canola and buttermilk with sugar and vanilla. Add egg and egg substitute, beating well after each addition. Stir in pumpkin. Add flour mixture alternately with sherry and blend well.

Pour into prepared loaf pan. Garnish top of loaf decoratively with pecan halves, if desired. Bake for 50 minutes, or until cake tester inserted in center comes out clean. Turn out onto wire rack to cool. Wrap and refrigerate until ready to slice.

Per serving: 240 calories, 43 g carbohydrate, 5.5 g fat, 1.5 g fiber, 4 g protein, 24 mg cholesterol, 210 mg sodium. *Calories from fat: 21%.*

Garden Sauté

Makes 4 servings.

1 tablespoon olive oil
2 zucchini, sliced
1 onion, cut in half, then sliced
1 clove garlic, minced or crushed, or 1/4 teaspoon garlic powder, or to taste

4 tomatoes, diced
$^3/_4$ teaspoon Italian seasoning, or to taste
Black pepper to taste
Salt to taste (optional)
$^1/_4$ cup light beer, wine, or broth

> Heat oil in large, nonstick frypan over medium heat. Add zucchini, onion, and garlic, and sauté for 3 minutes, stirring frequently. Add diced tomatoes, stir, and continue cooking. While cooking, sprinkle Italian seasoning, pepper and salt, if desired, over the top. Add beer, wine, or broth after tomato mixture has cooked a minute or so, and continue cooking and stirring until desired doneness (about two more minutes).

> **Per serving:** 89 calories, 12 g carbohydrate, 3.8 g fat, 3 g fiber, 2.7 g protein, 0 mg cholesterol, 16 mg sodium. *Calories from fat: 38%.*

High Mono Green Salad

Makes 6 servings.

1 avocado, cut into bite-size pieces
1 cucumber, sliced
$1^1/_2$ cups chopped tomatoes or cherry tomatoes cut in half
3 green onions, chopped (optional)
$1^1/_2$ cups canned garbanzo beans, drained and rinsed (optional)
12 tablespoons Wish-Bone Olive Oil Vinaigrette
8 cups (about 6 ounces) ready-to-serve salad greens of your choice

> Toss avocado, cucumber, tomatoes, onions, and garbanzo beans, if desired, together in serving bowl. Toss with dressing; set aside at room temperature or in refrigerator until needed.
> Right before mealtime, toss vegetable mixture with lettuce.

> **Per serving** (with beans): 143 (210) calories, 12 (23) g carbohydrate, 10.5 (11.5) g fat, 3.5 (5) g fiber, 3 (6) g protein, 0 mg cholesterol, 265 (300) mg sodium. *Calories from fat:* 66 (49)%.

Spinach and Blue Cheese Salad (with toasted almonds)

Makes 6 servings.

8 cups baby or regular spinach leaves (about 1 ready-to-serve package)
$1^1/_2$ cups canned kidney beans, drained and rinsed
2 ounces blue cheese or herbed feta cheese, crumbled

^{1}/$_3$ cup slivered almonds, toasted in nonstick cooking pan or microwave (heat, turning frequently, until almonds lightly brown)
^{3}/$_4$ cup Wish-Bone Olive Oil Vinaigrette

Just before serving, arrange spinach leaves in serving bowl or single-serving salad bowls. Toss spinach with kidney beans. Sprinkle cheese and almonds over the top. Drizzle vinaigrette over the top of serving bowl, or drizzle 2 tablespoons dressing over each individual salad bowl.

Per serving: 210 calories, 18.5 g carbohydrate, 11.2 g fat, 6 g fiber, 9.5 g protein, 7 mg cholesterol, 440 mg sodium. *Calories from fat:* 48%.

Saffron Rice

Makes 6 servings.

1^1/$_2$ tablespoons olive oil
3 tablespoons finely chopped onion
1^1/$_2$ cups long-grain rice
3 cups boiling water
1 teaspoon salt
^{1}/$_8$ teaspoon ground saffron

In a heavy 10- or 12-inch skillet, warm all over medium heat. Add onion and cook, stirring frequently, until it is soft and transparent (about 4 minutes). Pour in the rice and stir for 2 minutes to coat the rice with the oil. Add the boiling water, salt, and saffron. Bring mixture to boil, stirring frequently. Cover pan with lid and lower heat to a simmer. Cook undisturbed for 20 minutes. Rice should be tender with the water absorbed.

Per serving: 122 calories, 20 g carbohydrate, 3.5 g fat (mostly monounsaturated fats), .5 g fiber, 2 g protein, 357 sodium. *Calories from fat:* 26%.

SNACKS

Seven-Layer Mexican Dip

Makes dip for at least 6 hearty appetites.

16-ounce-can vegetarian refried beans or low-fat refried black beans
^{1}/$_2$ to 1 teaspoon chili powder
Black pepper to taste

Jalapeño sauce (green or red, mild or hot) to taste
³/₄ cup fat-free or light sour cream
1 avocado, mashed
1 tablespoon low-fat mayonnaise
1¹/₂ teaspoons lemon juice
1 cup grated reduced-fat sharp cheddar cheese
1 cup finely chopped tomatoes
5 green onions, chopped
2 ounces black olives, chopped

Suggested dippers
Low-fat or reduced-fat tortilla chips
Soft flour tortillas cut into triangles
Celery or carrot sticks

Heat beans in small saucepan over low heat until warm and softened. Stir in chili powder, pepper, and jalapeño sauce. Pour into 8-by-8-inch baking pan or casserole dish (or similar), spread over bottom, and let cool. Spread sour cream over the top of beans. In small bowl or small food processor, blend avocado with mayonnaise and lemon juice. Spread guacamole evenly over sour cream. Top with grated cheese. Sprinkle chopped tomatoes evenly over the top. Sprinkle tomatoes with green onions and olives. Refrigerate until needed. Serve with suggested dippers.

Per serving of dip: 213 calories, 20 g carbohydrate, 9.5 g fat, 6 g fiber, 11 g protein, 11 mg cholesterol, 503 mg sodium. *Calories from fat: 40%.*

Easy Roasted Potatoes

Makes 5 servings.

4 teaspoons olive oil
¹/₂ teaspoon garlic powder
¹/₂ teaspoon fines herbes or Italian seasoning
5 medium potatoes (7 to 8 small potatoes), cut into chunks and cooked in microwave on High for 12 to 15 minutes, until tender
Nonstick cooking spray

Preheat oven to 500° or turn on broiler. Mix first three ingredients together in medium-size bowl or large Ziploc storage bag. Add potato pieces and toss with seasoning mixture. Keep turning potato pieces around until all pieces are evenly coated with seasoning. Coat a jelly-roll pan with nonstick cooking spray. Spread potatoes evenly on a prepared pan. Bake or broil until lightly brown. (If baking, cooking

time is around 10 minutes, if broiling, cooking time is a few minutes—watching carefully.)

> **Per serving:** 250 calories, 51 g carbohydrate, 3.8 g fat, 5 g fiber, 5 g
> protein, 0 mg cholesterol, 16 mg sodium. *Calories from fat:* 13.6%.

Quick French Onion Dip

Makes five ¹/₄-cup servings.

¹/₂ package (3 tablespoons) Knorr French Onion Soup and Recipe Mix
1¹/₈ cups fat-free sour cream
1 tablespoon real mayonnaise
3 tablespoons low-fat or light mayonnaise

> Stir soup mix, sour cream, mayonnaise, and low-fat mayonnaise until
> blended. Cover and chill. Stir before serving.

> **Per serving:** 105 calories, 12 g carbohydrate, 4 g fat, 0 g fiber, 3 g
> protein, 4 mg cholesterol, 390 mg sodium. *Calories from fat:* 35%.

ENTRÉES

Oat Bran Pizza

Makes about 6 servings, 2 slices each.

This recipe is better than it sounds! Borrow a friend's bread machine for
this recipe, if you don't have one.

1 cup plus 2 tablespoons water
2 tablespoons olive oil or canola oil
1 cup oat bran
2¹/₃ cups plus 1 tablespoon, if needed, bread flour or regular flour
2 tablespoons grated Parmesan, if desired
1¹/₂ teaspoons Italian seasoning, if desired
1 teaspoon sugar
1 teaspoon salt
2¹/₂ teaspoons bread machine yeast

Topping
1 cup favorite bottled spaghetti sauce, or tomato sauce blended with 1
    teaspoon Italian seasoning and 2 cloves minced garlic
4 ounces reduced-fat sharp cheddar (or similar), grated
4 ounces part-skim mozzarella, grated
Assorted vegetable toppings (onions, peppers, mushrooms), if desired

50% less-fat salami (Gallo), if desired
70% less-fat pepperoni (Hormel), if desired

Measure carefully, placing all crust ingredients in bread machine pan in the order recommended by the manufacturer. Select Dough/Manual cycle (in my bread maker this takes 1 hour and 40 minutes). Check dough after first 5 minutes to see if another tablespoon of flour is needed for proper dough texture.

Preheat oven to 400°. After dough cycle, divide dough in half and dust each half generously with flour. Pat dough into two 15-inch-diameter pizza pans or press each half into a circle on two cookie sheets. Spread sauce evenly over the crust. Sprinkle cheese evenly over the top. Add other toppings, if desired.

Bake 18 to 20 minutes, or until crust is light brown and cheese is bubbly.

Per serving (includes all ingredients except the last three, which are optional): 375 calories, 52 g carbohydrate, 12.5 g fat, 4.5 g fiber, 19 g protein, 20 mg cholesterol, 785 mg sodium. *Calories from fat:* 30%.

Variation: Before adding the grated cheese, add 1 skinless roasted chicken breast, shredded into bite-size pieces, and 1/2 cup of kidney beans to each pizza. One serving (two slices) of this pizza will be 458 calories, 59 g carbohydrate, 14 g fat, 7.5 g fiber, 30 g protein, 45 mg cholesterol, 807 mg sodium.

Oat Bran Bread

Makes 1 large loaf, 14 slices.

This bread is delicious fresh out of the bread machine. I love it without anything on it! It makes great sandwiches or toast. I had a difficult time finding oat bran bread in supermarkets where I live, so I thought a bread machine recipe would be essential for bread lovers across the country. If you don't have a bread machine, see if you can borrow one to make this bread. If you find that you really like it and it helps reduce your blood glucose response after eating bread, you might then decide to invest in a bread machine of your own. The recipe is based on using a 2-pound bread machine.

1 cup plus 2 tablespoons low-fat milk
2 tablespoons canola oil
1 tablespoon honey
1/4 cup pancake syrup

1 large egg
2¹/₄ cups bread flour
¹/₂ cup whole wheat flour
³/₄ cup oat bran
¹/₂ cup old-fashioned oats
1¹/₂ teaspoons salt
2¹/₂ teaspoons bread machine yeast or active dry yeast

Place all the ingredients (preferably at room temperature) in the machine in the order listed (add salt to one corner of the machine while adding the yeast in the center of the flour after making a small hole for it with your finger). Set machine for basic white bread or wheat bread and press Start or On.

Per 2-slice serving: 322 calories, 58.5 g carbohydrate, 7 g fat, 4 g fiber, 11 g protein, 32 mg cholesterol, 495 mg sodium. *Calories from fat: 20%.*

Antipasto Sandwich

Makes 1 sandwich.

1 kaiser bun (about 67 grams), or a foccacia bun or wedge, or 2 slices oat bran bread
5 slices light salami (turkey, pork, and beef) with 50% less fat
1 ounce reduced-fat cheese of your choice (part-skim mozzarella, reduced-fat sharp cheddar, Monterey jack, or part-skim Jarlsberg), sliced thin
¹/₄ avocado, peeled and sliced
3 tomato slices or 2 pieces roasted red pepper (available in jars in some supermarkets)
Dijon mustard or olive oil (optional)

Cut kaiser or foccacia bun in half. Lay salami slices evenly on one half of the bread, and top with cheese slices, avocado slices, then tomato or red pepper slices. Spread other half of bread with Dijon mustard or brush with olive oil, if desired. Put two halves together.

Per sandwich: 427 calories, 43.5 g carbohydrate, 19.5 g fat, 3 g fiber, 21 g protein, 40 mg cholesterol, 1,000 mg sodium. *Calories from fat: 41%.*

Quick and Crustless Vegetable Quiche

Makes 8 servings.

Nonstick cooking spray
2 stalks broccoli, cut into small pieces

8 mushrooms, sliced
3/4 cup chopped onions
2 cloves garlic, minced or crushed
Broth or water (optional)
3/4 teaspoon oregano
3/4 teaspoon basil
6 eggs
1 1/2 cups egg substitute
Approximately 1/2 cup low-fat milk
4 ounces reduced-fat sharp cheddar, grated
4 ounces reduced-fat Monterey jack or Swiss cheese, grated

Preheat oven to 350°. Coat a 10-inch pie plate with nonstick cooking spray. Sauté broccoli, mushrooms, onions, and garlic in large nonstick frypan coated generously with nonstick cooking spray. Add broth or water if moisture is needed during cooking. Add oregano and basil, and cook until just tender. Add eggs and egg substitute to 4-cup measure. Add milk until mixture equals 3 1/2 cups (about 1/2 cup of milk). Add egg mixture to mixing bowl and beat until blended.

Spread half of the grated cheese in the bottom of pan. Add vegetable mixture. Top with rest of cheese. Pour egg mixture gently over and bake for 40 minutes, or until set.

Per serving: 180 calories, 5 g carbohydrate, 9 g fat, 2 g fiber, 19 g protein, 174 mg cholesterol, 295 mg sodium. *Calories from fat: 45%.*

Chicken Prosciutto

Makes 8 small or 4 large servings.

If you can't find Fontina in your local supermarket or specialty store, you can substitute reduced-fat Monterey jack or Swiss cheese.

4 chicken breast halves, skinless and boneless
Freshly ground black pepper
Flour
4 teaspoons canola oil
Nonstick cooking spray
8 thin slices prosciutto
4 ounces Fontina, thinly sliced or shredded
1 1/2 tablespoons Parmesan, freshly grated
4 tablespoons chicken broth
3 cups steamed rice or cooked spaghetti (6 ounces uncooked)

Preheat oven to 350°. With a sharp knife, carefully slice each chicken breast in half horizontally to make 8 thin slices. Lay them an inch or so apart on a long strip of wax paper and cover with another strip of wax paper. Pound the chicken lightly with flat side of a cleaver or bottom of a heavy bottle. Strip off paper. Season with fresh pepper. Dip each breast in flour and shake off excess.

In a large, nonstick frypan, heat oil over moderate heat (spread oil with spatula to coat pan evenly). If you are using a medium-size frypan, fry 4 chicken pieces at a time using 2 teaspoons of oil and repeat with remaining chicken and oil. Sauté chicken to a light golden brown. Transfer chicken to a 9-by-13-inch baking pan that has been coated with nonstick cooking spray. Place a slice of prosciutto on each piece of chicken and then top each with a slice of cheese or $1/4$ cup grated cheese. Sprinkle with Parmesan and drizzle chicken broth over the tops. Bake uncovered for 10 to 15 minutes, or until cheese is melted and lightly browned. Serve each chicken piece over $1/3$ cup spaghetti or steamed rice.

> **Per small serving** (including spaghetti or rice): 260 calories, 25 g carbohydrate, 10 g fat, .5 g fiber, 23.5 g protein, 66 mg cholesterol, 432 mg sodium. *Calories from fat:* 34%.

Chicken and Cabbage Ramen Salad

Makes 6 servings.

Try to find the Nissan brand of ramen noodles, which has 7 grams fat per serving for some of its flavors; other brands have 8 grams. If you are able to find Campbell's Low Fat Ramen, it will reduce the fat by about 1 gram per serving of salad.

$1/4$ cup slivered almonds
3 tablespoons sesame seeds
Nonstick cooking spray
10 packages shredded cabbage, 4 to 6 cups, or $1/2$ head of cabbage, shredded
4 to 6 green onions, finely chopped
1 small can sliced water chestnuts, drained and rinsed
2 cooked skinless chicken breasts, cut or shredded into bite-size pieces

Dressing
3 tablespoons olive oil
$1^1/2$ teaspoons sesame oil
$1/4$ cup apple or orange juice

2 tablespoons honey
1/3 cup rice vinegar
2 teaspoons Wondra quick-mixing flour, or cornstarch
Top Ramen seasoning packet
1/4 teaspoon pepper
1 package (3 ounces) Top Ramen noodles, chicken, chicken vegetable, or
  Oriental flavor, crumbled into small pieces

Add almonds and sesame seeds to a glass measure that has been
coated at the bottom with nonstick cooking spray. Microwave mixture
on High for 2 to 3 minutes, stirring after each minute, until almonds
are brown. You can also heat almonds and sesame seeds in a nonstick
frypan over medium heat, stirring frequently, until nuts and seeds are
light brown.

After nut mixture has cooled, add to serving bowl along with
cabbage, green onions, water chestnuts, and chicken. Prepare dressing
by adding all dressing ingredients to small food processor or blender
(or stir well by hand) and process until well blended.

Just before serving, toss cabbage and chicken mixture with ramen
noodles and dressing.

Per serving: 286 calories, 22 g carbohydrate, 16.0 g fat, 3 g fiber, 13.5
g protein, 24 mg cholesterol, 298 mg sodium. *Calories from fat: 50%.*

Mexican Pizza

Makes 6 servings.

1 pound ground beef (10 percent fat)
2 tablespoons Lawry's taco seasoning
Nonstick cooking spray
6 flour tortillas
16-ounce-can no-fat refried beans
1 1/2 cups (6 ounces) grated reduced-fat sharp cheddar or Monterey jack
Picante sauce or salsa (optional)

Preheat oven to 350°. Brown ground beef. Stir in taco seasoning. Coat
a deep casserole dish or pie plate with nonstick cooking spray. Lay
one tortilla in dish. Spread half the beef mixture over the tortilla. Top
with another tortilla and coat top with nonstick cooking spray. Spread
half of beans over the top. Place tortilla on top and coat with nonstick
cooking spray. Top with tortilla and coat with nonstick cooking spray.
Spread half of cheese over tortilla. Repeat layers with remaining beef,
beans, cheese, and tortillas.

Bake in preheated oven for 30 minutes. Serve with picante sauce or salsa, if desired.

Per serving: 373 calories, 40 g carbohydrate, 12 g fat, 7 g fiber, 26 g protein, 36 mg cholesterol, 880 mg sodium. *Calories from fat: 29%.*

Super Quick Pesto Pasta

Makes 4 servings.

5 cups drained spaghetti (10 ounces uncooked), cooked al dente
4 ounces ($^1/_2$ cup) prepared pesto made with olive or canola oil (such as Armanino)
2 cups vegetables, such as broccoli and sliced carrots

Place hot spaghetti in a warmed pasta serving dish. Add pesto and 1 or 2 tablespoons pasta cooking water. Steam or microwave vegetables only until crisp-tender. Add to pasta and pesto, and toss together. Serve immediately.

Per serving: 370 calories, 57 g carbohydrate, 10 g fat, 5 g fiber, 12 g protein, 5 mg cholesterol, 222 mg sodium. *Calories from fat: 25%.*

Soluble Fiber Meat Loaf

Makes 5 servings.

1$^1/_4$ cup canned chick-peas, drained and rinsed
$^1/_2$ cup rolled oats
$^1/_2$ teaspoon black pepper
$^1/_2$ teaspoon salt (optional)
2 cloves garlic, minced or pressed, or $^1/_2$ teaspoon garlic powder
1 tablespoon Worcestershire sauce
2 tablespoons Heinz chili sauce
1 tablespoon prepared mustard
1 pound ground sirloin (about 9 percent fat)
1 cup grated reduced-fat sharp cheddar (optional)
1 small onion, finely chopped
Nonstick cooking spray
1 cup tomato sauce

Preheat oven to 350°. Add first eight ingredients to mixer or food processor (or mash with pastry blender or potato masher) and process until well mixed (there will still be some lumps). If using a mixer, add beef, cheese, and onion, and mix until well blended. If using a food processor, blend bean mixture with beef, cheese, and onion with hands or a spoon in a large mixing bowl.

Coat a 9-by-5-inch loaf pan with nonstick cooking spray. Add beef mixture to pan and form into a loaf. Bake 30 minutes. Pour tomato sauce over the top and bake 15 minutes longer.

Per serving (including cheese): 256 (320) calories, 25 g carbohydrate, 8 (11.8) g fat, 4.5 g fiber, 21.5 (28) g protein, 25 (37) mg cholesterol, 500 (620) mg sodium. *Calories from fat:* 28 (33) %.

Beef Tacos

Makes 2 tacos each.

1 pound ground beef (9% fat)
$^1/_2$ cup finely chopped onion
$^1/_2$ to 1 packet taco seasoning
$^2/_3$ cup water
4 teaspoons canola oil
8 large corn tortillas
1 cup chopped tomatoes
2 cups shredded lettuce
1 cup grated reduced-fat Monterey jack or sharp cheddar, or mixture

Brown beef with chopped onion in large nonstick frypan. Add taco seasoning and water, and let simmer about 5 minutes.

In another large nonstick frypan, heat $^1/_2$ teaspoon of canola oil in center of pan over medium heat. Add corn tortilla and, using a spatula, spread the tortilla around the center of the pan to distribute the oil. Flip it over frequently to heat both sides. Once the tortilla starts to stiffen (about 2 minutes), place it on paper towels and fold it over into a taco shape. Repeat with remaining oil and tortillas.

Serve beef filling with taco shells, tomatoes, lettuce, cheese, and sour cream and salsa if desired.

Per serving: 393 calories, 28 g carbohydrate, 15.75 g fat, 5 g fiber, 27 g protein, 47 mg cholesterol, 220 mg sodium. *Calories from fat:* 36%.

Variation: Use $^3/_4$ pound ground beef and 1 cup of canned black or pinto beans to lower the fat and cholesterol a little and increase the fiber. 2 tacos made this way contain 403 calories, 27 g protein, 37 g carbohydrate, 14 g fat, 37 mg cholesterol. *Calories from fat:* 32%.

Simple Salmon Pasta Salad

Makes about 3 servings.

3 cups bow tie or rotelle pasta, cooked al dente
1 cup salmon flakes (freshly cooked or grilled salmon fillets or steaks,
    broken into flakes with fork, with no bones or skin)
1 cup crisp-tender asparagus pieces, steamed or microwaved
3 green onions, finely chopped

Dressing
1 tablespoon mayonnaise
3 tablespoons low-fat mayonnaise
1 tablespoon lemon juice
1$\frac{1}{2}$ teaspoons Dijon or prepared mustard
$\frac{1}{2}$ teaspoon dill weed
Black pepper to taste

Place first four ingredients in serving bowl. Blend dressing ingredients in a 1- or 2-cup measure until smooth. Add to pasta salad ingredients and stir to mix.

Per serving: 382 calories, 47 g carbohydrate, 11.5 g fat, 4 g fiber, 22 g protein, 33 mg cholesterol, 205 mg sodium. *Calories from fat: 27%.*

Chinese Chicken Salad

Makes 4 large servings.

You can usually find wonton wraps in the produce department next to the tofu.

4 skinless chicken breast halves
Orange juice or low-sodium soy sauce
11-ounce can mandarin orange slices, drained
$\frac{1}{3}$ cup green onions, sliced diagonally, with part of green
Nonstick cooking spray
10 wonton wraps, cut in 1/8-inch strips
Canola nonstick cooking spray
1 head iceberg lettuce
3 tablespoons slivered almonds

Dressing
2 tablespoons low-sodium soy sauce
$\frac{1}{4}$ cup orange juice
2 tablespoons sugar (optional), or 1 packet of Equal or Sweet 'n Low
1 teaspoon prepared mustard

1 tablespoon sesame oil
3 tablespoons rice vinegar
$^1/_4$ teaspoon five-spice powder (optional)

Toast slivered almonds by cooking over medium heat in a nonstick frypan until lightly browned, stirring frequently. Set aside.

Grill or broil chicken breasts, basting with orange juice or soy sauce. Cut diagonally to make decorative strips. Toss chicken with orange slices and onions in serving bowl.

For oven-baked wonton strips, preheat oven to 375°. Coat a baking sheet with nonstick cooking spray. Place strips in single layer on baking sheet. Spray tops with nonstick cooking spray. Bake 10 to 15 minutes, or until lightly browned.

Mix dressing ingredients in small bowl until well blended or use small food processor to combine ingredients. Pour dressing over chicken mixture and toss. Right before serving, thinly shred lettuce, and toss with chicken mixture. Divide among 4 dinner plates; sprinkle each serving with almonds and wonton strips.

Per serving: 312 calories, 25 g carbohydrate, 8.7 g fat, 3 g fiber, 33 g protein, 70 mg cholesterol, 725 mg sodium. *Calories from fat: 25%.*

Salade Niçoise

Makes 6 servings.

3 medium potatoes, cooked, cubed, and chilled
3 hard-boiled eggs, quartered, yolks discarded, and chilled
2 medium tomatoes, quartered
One 13-ounce can solid white tuna, in water, drained
6$^1/_2$-ounce jar marinated artichoke hearts, drained
1 cup (8$^3/_4$-ounce can) kidney beans, drained and rinsed
$^1/_2$ cup Greek, Spinach, or black olives (pitted or stuffed with pimiento), about 18 olives

Dressing
3 tablespoons olive oil
$^1/_4$ cup red wine vinegar
$^1/_3$ cup apple juice
2 tablespoons honey
$^1/_2$ teaspoon salt (optional)
$^1/_8$ teaspoon pepper
$^1/_2$ teaspoon chervil
$^1/_2$ teaspoon tarragon
8 cups lettuce of your choice

Place potatoes and egg whites in medium-size serving bowl. Add tomatoes. Separate tuna into bite-size pieces and add to serving bowl along with the artichoke hearts, beans, and olives.

Place all dressing ingredients in a small food processor or blender; process until well blended and smooth. Pour into serving bowl and toss well with tuna, eggs, and vegetables. Place about 1¹/₃ cups of lettuce on each plate. Divide the tuna mixture into six even portions and spoon over lettuce.

Per serving: 342 calories, 43 g carbohydrate, 10 g fat, 8 g fiber, 22 g protein, 15 mg cholesterol, 695 mg sodium (517, if no salt is used in the dressing). *Calories from fat:* 26%.

Salmon Burgers

Makes 2 servings.

6-ounce can skinless, boneless pink salmon in spring water, drained, or the
    boneless, skinless cooked meat from 1 large (8 ounces) salmon steak
1 tablespoon chopped onion
1¹/₂ teaspoons diced dill pickle
1 tablespoon low-fat mayonnaise
¹/₂ teaspoon mustard
1 small clove garlic
1¹/₂ teaspoons lemon juice
2 to 3 tablespoons seasoned bread crumbs (or other bread
    crumbs)
Canola nonstick cooking spray
2 hamburger buns (optional)
Lettuce (optional)
Sliced tomato (optional)

Blend the above ingredients together in bowl with a fork until well mixed. Form with clean hands into 2 hamburger-size salmon patties. Heat a nonstick frypan over medium heat. Spray with canola nonstick cooking spray. Add patties and cook a couple minutes on both sides, or until both sides are lightly browned. Serve on a bun with lettuce and sliced tomato, if desired.

Per serving (with bun): 183 (312) calories, 11 (33) g carbohydrate, 7.3 (9.7) g fat, 5 (2) g protein, 18 (22) g protein, 49 mg cholesterol, 397 (649) mg sodium. *Calories from fat:* 36 (28) percent.

Ranch Vegetable Chicken Salad

Makes 4 servings.

1/4 envelope Original Hidden Valley Ranch Party Dip
1/2 cup nonfat sour cream
2 teaspoons light or low-fat mayonnaise
2 green onions, chopped
2 celery stalks, thinly sliced
1 carrot, grated
1/2 red bell pepper, chopped
3 skinless, boneless chicken breasts, cooked, cooled, and shredded into
    bite-size pieces
Lettuce (optional)
Approximately 8 slices bread of choice (optional)

In medium-size serving bowl, blend ranch dip powder with sour cream and mayonnaise. Stir in green onions, celery, carrot, red pepper, and chicken pieces. Serve with lettuce or bread, if desired.

Per serving: 168 calories, 9 g carbohydrate, 4 g fat, 1 g fiber, 22 g protein, 56 mg cholesterol, 317 mg sodium. *Calories from fat: 23%.*

Quick-Fix Schilling Chili

Makes four 1-cup servings.

This chili is excellent served with Oat Bran Corn Bread.

1 pound ground sirloin or ground turkey breast (or half and half)
1 packet (1 1/4 oz.) Schilling Chili Seasoning
16-ounce can low-sodium chopped stewed tomatoes
15-ounce can low-sodium kidney beans, drained and rinsed
1/2 cup grated reduced-fat sharp cheddar or Monterey jack

Brown ground beef or turkey in large saucepan or covered frypan, breaking into small pieces as it cooks. Stir in seasoning packet, stewed tomatoes, and kidney beans. Bring to a boil, cover, and simmer 10 minutes. Spoon into soup bowls and sprinkle cheese over the top.

Per serving: 294 calories, 29 g carbohydrate, 8.5 g fat, 10 g fiber, 25 g protein, 31 mgs cholesterol, 391 mg sodium. *Calories from fat: 26%.*

Chicken-Mango-Avocado Salad

Makes 3 chicken-salad servings.

3 cooked skinless chicken breasts, roasted or barbecued
1 mango, peeled, seed removed
³/₄ avocado, peeled and pitted
3 green onions, finely chopped
1 cup chopped tomato (any type)

Dressing
1 tablespoon mayonnaise
1 tablespoon fat-free sour cream
2 tablespoons orange juice
Freshly ground black pepper to taste (optional)

Cut chicken into bite-size pieces. Cut mango flesh into bite-size pieces. Cut avocado into bite-size pieces. Add chicken, mango, and avocado to medium-size serving bowl. Stir in green onions and tomatoes.

In a small bowl, blend dressing ingredients well. Drizzle over salad ingredients and stir to blend.

Per serving: 327 calories, 21 g carbohydrate, 14.9 g fat (mostly monounsaturated and polyunsaturated fat), 5 g fiber, 29 g protein, 75 mg cholesterol, 110 mg sodium. *Calories from fat:* 40%.

Note: Most people prefer the taste of real mayonnaise; however, if you like light or fat-free mayonnaise, go ahead and use it. If you use light mayonnaise instead of the regular, a serving will contain 311 calories, 13 g fat (mostly from monounsatured and polyunsaturated fat), and 73 mg cholesterol.

DESSERTS

Light Chocolate Cake

Makes 14 slices.

You've heard of mayonnaise cake. Well, get ready for Wesson Oil cake. This is a family recipe submitted by Debra Mulanax of Walnut Creek. Her family has been making this cake for years. As a nutritionist I liked this recipe for two reasons. First, it uses oil, so I can use canola oil (luckily Wesson makes a canola oil) and produce a cake with almost no saturated fat (and mostly monounsaturated fats). Second, it calls for baking chocolate, and I can easily use cocoa in its place by using the standard conversion of 3 level tablespoons of cocoa plus 1 tablespoon oil equals 1 ounce of baking chocolate.

Of course, at this point my work has only just begun. I reduced the cup of oil called for to $^1/_4$ cup and replaced the lost oil with chocolate syrup and fat-free cream cheese. I needed to use chocolate syrup as a partial replacement for the fat because after making it for the first time, even using the baking chocolate, it needed a stronger chocolate flavor.

I also replaced two of the eggs called for with fat-free egg substitute or egg whites. I doubled the amount of vanilla and used a lower-fat milk.

I made so many changes in this recipe Debra and her family probably wouldn't recognize it if they saw it—but would they recognize the new and nutritionally improved chocolate cake taste? That's for me to know and you to find out—just kidding. I ran a sample of the cake over to Debra and it was a hit. This cake is particularly great for people who are really concerned with lowering their saturated fat by boosting their monounsaturated fats. Before the low-fat makeover, a serving of this recipe contained 335 calories, 20 grams of fat, and 48 milligrams of cholesterol (not including frosting!)

Nonstick cooking spray
6 tablespoons chocolate syrup
6 tablespoons fat-free cream cheese
$^1/_2$ cup high-quality cocoa
1 egg, lightly beaten
5 tablespoons canola oil
1 cup sugar
$^1/_3$ cup fat-free egg substitute
2 teaspoons vanilla
2 cups flour
4 teaspoons baking powder
$^1/_2$ teaspoon salt
1 cup 1-percent low-fat milk, or similar

Preheat oven to 350°. Generously coat a 10-inch tube pan, or two 9-inch layer cake pans, with nonstick cooking spray. Place chocolate syrup and cream cheese in a mixing bowl and beat until blended. Blend in cocoa on the lowest speed.

Add egg and canola oil to mixing bowl and beat until blended. Add sugar, egg substitute, and vanilla, and beat until smooth.

Mix flour, baking powder, and salt in separate bowl. Add half the flour mixture to chocolate batter. Then blend in half the milk. Add the remaining flour mixture and milk, alternately. Beat until smooth. Bake about 40 minutes for tube pan, or until cake tests done, or 30 minutes for layer cake pans.

Per serving: 211 calories, 37 g carbohydrates, 6 g fat, 2 g fiber, 5 g protein, 16 mg cholesterol, 254 mg sodium. *Calories from fat: 25%.*

Frozen Light Lemon Pie

Makes 8 servings.

1 packet Dream Whip powder
$1/2$ cup cold 1-percent low-fat milk
$1/2$ teaspoon vanilla
Two 6-ounce containers Yoplait Light Lemon Cream Pie yogurt
Zest from 1 lemon, finely chopped
$1^1/2$ cups Light Cool Whip
4 drops yellow food coloring (optional)
1 Keebler Reduced-Fat Graham Cracker Ready Crust

Add Dream Whip powder, milk, and vanilla to mixing bowl. Beat on high until topping thickens and forms peaks (4 to 6 minutes). Gently stir in yogurt, lemon zest, Cool Whip, and yellow food coloring, if desired, until well blended. Spoon mixture into crust. Freeze 4 hours or overnight until firm. Let stand in refrigerator 15 minutes or until pie can be cut easily. Store leftover pie in freezer.

Per serving: 162 calories, 24 g carbohydrate, 4 g fat, <1g fiber, 3 g protein, 1 mg cholesterol, 120 mg sodium. *Calories from fat: 22%.*

Apple-Oat Crisp

Makes 9 large servings.

Nonstick cooking spray
6 to 8 cups sliced apples
$3/4$ cup flour
$3/4$ cup old-fashioned oats
$1/2$ cup firmly packed dark brown sugar
4 packets Sweet 'n Low
$1/2$ teaspoon salt
$3/4$ teaspoon cinnamon
$1/4$ teaspoon allspice
4 tablespoons butter or margarine, melted
1 teaspoon vanilla

1 to 2 tablespoons buttermilk or whole or low-fat milk
Light vanilla ice cream

Preheat oven to 375°. Coat 9-by-9-inch baking dish with nonstick cooking spray. Place apple slices into prepared dish. In medium-size bowl, blend the dry ingredients. Drizzle butter, vanilla, and 1 tablespoon of buttermilk over the top and blend with fork until the mixture is crumbly. Add one more tablespoon of buttermilk, if needed, for desired crumbly texture. Sprinkle crumb mixture evenly over the fruit.

Bake for 30 to 35 minutes, or until apples are tender and top is lightly browned. Makes 9 large servings. Serve warm with light vanilla ice cream, if desired.

Per serving: 190 calories, 33 g carbohydrate, 6 g fat, 4 g fiber, 3 g protein, 14 mg cholesterol, 176 mg sodium. *Calories from fat: 27%.*

Variation: You can use 4 cups of boysenberries instead of apples; each serving will have 170 calories, 27 g carbohydrate instead of the above.

Choc-Oat-Chip Bars

Makes 24 bars.

$^1/_2$ cup butter or margarine, softened '
$^1/_2$ cup fat-free cream cheese
$1^1/_4$ cups firmly packed brown sugar
$^1/_4$ cup light pancake syrup
1 egg
$^1/_4$ cup egg substitute
2 tablespoons milk
1 tablespoon vanilla
$1^3/_4$ cups all-purpose flour
1 teaspoon baking soda
$^1/_2$ teaspoon salt (optional)
$2^1/_2$ cups Quaker Oats (quick or old-fashioned, uncooked)
1 cup (6 ounces) semisweet chocolate chips
Nonstick cooking spray

Preheat oven to 375°. Beat butter with cream cheese. Add brown sugar and beat until creamy. Add egg, egg substitute, milk, and vanilla; beat well. Mix flour, baking soda, and salt together. Add to moist ingredients and blend well. Stir in oats and chocolate chips; mix well. Press dough onto bottom of 13-by-9-inch baking pan that has been coated with nonstick cooking spray. Bake 20 minutes. Let cool in pan. Cut into 24 bars.

Per serving: 176 calories, 26 g carbohydrate, 6.7 g fat, 2 g fiber, 4 g protein, 20 mg cholesterol, 133 mg sodium. *Calories from fat:* 34%.

Variation: To make Peanut Butter Choc-Oat-Chip Bars, just use ¹/₂ cup creamy peanut butter in place of the butter or margarine. Each serving will then have 173 calories, 5 g protein, 27 g carbohydrate, 5.4 g fat, 9 mg cholesterol, 120 mg sodium, 2 g fiber. *Calories from fat:* 28%.

Very Berry Ice Cream

Makes about 6 half-cup servings.

3 cups 1% or 2% low-fat milk
¹/₂ cup sugar
8 packets Equal (NutraSweet)
About 3 cups fresh or frozen and thawed unsweetened boysenberries or
    strawberries, to make 1¹/₂ cups pureed
2 cups Lite Cool Whip

Prepare ice cream maker according to manufacturer's directions. In a large mixing bowl, combine all ingredients. Add to ice cream maker and freeze into ice cream according to manufacturer's directions.

Per serving: 100 calories, 20 g carbohydrate, 1.5 g fat, 1.5 g fiber, 2 g protein, 5 mg cholesterol, 38 mg sodium. *Calories from fat:* 12%.

Strawberry Shortcake

Makes 6 servings.

2 pints strawberries, sliced
6 to 8 packets Equal or Sweet 'n Low
2¹/₃ cups Reduced Fat Bisquick Baking Mix
¹/₂ cup 1% or 2% low-fat milk
1 tablespoon canola oil
2 tablespoons corn syrup
Light whipped cream, Light Cool Whip, or Dream Whip (optional)

Add strawberries to medium-size serving bowl and sprinkle with Equal; let stand 1 hour. Heat oven to 425°. Stir Bisquick, milk, oil, and corn syrup together in a large bowl until soft dough forms. Knead 8 or so times on lightly floured cutting board. Roll dough into ¹/₂-inch-thick round.

Cut with 3-inch biscuit cutter. Place on ungreased cookie sheet. Bake 10 to 12 minutes, or until golden brown. Split shortcakes and fill and top with strawberries. Top with a dollop of light whipped cream, or Cool Whip or Dream Whip, if desired.

Per serving: 261 calories, 47 g carbohydrate, 6 g fat, 3 g fiber, 6 g protein, 1 mg cholesterol, 557 mg sodium. *Calories from fat:* 20%. Two tablespoons of pressurized light whipped cream will add 20 calories, 2 g fat, 1 g saturated fat, and 5 mg cholesterol to each serving.

Cocoa Brownies

Makes about 24 brownies.

Nonstick cooking spray
$1/3$ cup fat-free sour cream
$1/4$ cup canola oil
$1/4$ cup chocolate syrup
1 cup sugar
2 tablespoons water or strong coffee
1 egg
$1/4$ cup fat-free egg substitute
1 tablespoon vanilla
$3/4$ cup cocoa
$1 1/3$ cups all-purpose flour
$1/2$ teaspoon baking powder
$1/4$ teaspoon salt
Powdered sugar or $1/4$ cup white chocolate chips (optional)

Preheat oven to 350° (325° for a glass baking dish). Coat a 9-by-13-inch baking pan with nonstick cooking spray.

Place sour cream in a mixing bowl and beat at low speed. Slowly add oil, chocolate syrup, sugar, and water or coffee. Add egg, egg substitute, and vanilla, and beat just until blended. Combine cocoa, flour, baking powder, and salt in a bowl; beat quickly into sugar mixture. Pour batter into prepared pan and spread it evenly. Bake in center of oven for 10 minutes or until wooden pick inserted in center comes out slightly sticky. If you like cakey brownies, bake a couple of minutes more. Cool in pan. Use a flour sifter to dust brownies with powdered sugar, if desired. You could also drizzle the top of brownies with melted white chocolate chips (microwave $1/4$ cup of chips in microwave-safe small dish on the Defrost setting for about 90 seconds). Cut into 24 bars.

Per serving: 93 calories, 16 g carbohydrate, 2.8 g fat, 1 g fiber, 2 g protein, 8 mg cholesterol, 65 mg sodium. *Calories from fat:* 27%.

Soft Chocolate Chip Cookies

Makes 36 cookies.

Nonstick cooking spray
$1/2$ cup butter, softened
$1/2$ cup nonfat cream cheese
$1/2$ cup granulated sugar
$3/4$ cup firmly packed brown sugar
6 to 8 packets Equal (NutraSweet)
$1/2$ cup fat-free egg substitute
2 teaspoons vanilla
2 cups flour
$2^1/2$ cups old-fashioned oats
$1/2$ teaspoon salt
1 teaspoon baking powder
1 teaspoon baking soda
$1^1/2$ cups semisweet chocolate chips

Preheat oven to 350° and coat cookie sheets with nonstick cooking spray.

Cream butter with cream cheese in mixer bowl. Add sugars and sugar substitute, and beat until blended. Add egg substitute and vanilla, beating well.

Combine flour, oats, salt, baking powder, and baking soda in large food processor, or mix together and process small amounts in a blender and process for about 8 seconds. Combine flour mixture with wet ingredients just until blended. Add chocolate chips. Shape dough into 1-inch-diameter balls with a scoop or a tablespoon, and place on cookie sheets. Spray bottom of flat-bottomed glass with nonstick cooking spray. Press gently onto cookie dough for flatter cookies (you will need to respray the bottom of the glass every 2 or 3 cookies). Bake about 9 minutes, or until lightly browned. Let cool on wire rack.

Per serving (1 cookie): 130 calories, 20 g carbohydrate, 5 g fat 1 g fiber, 3 g protein, 7 mg cholesterol, 133 mg sodium. *Calories from fat:* 34%.

Blender Chocolate Mousse

Makes 5 servings.

$1/4$ cup water
1 packet unflavored gelatin
$3/4$ cup semisweet chocolate chips

$^1/_2$ cup egg substitute
$^1/_2$ cup fat-free cream cheese
$^1/_3$ cup cocoa
2 to 3 teaspoons Grand Marnier or other liqueur
1 cup scalded 1% or 2% low-fat milk

Add $^1/_4$ cup water to small saucepan. Sprinkle gelatin over the top and let stand a few minutes. Heat mixture over low heat, stirring, until dissolved (about 4 minutes).

Place chocolate chips, egg substitute, cream cheese, cocoa, liqueur, and gelatin mixture in blender container. Cover and blend on lowest speed for 5 seconds. Pour in the scalded milk. Cover and blend on high speed 2 to 3 minutes. Pour into 5 individual serving dishes. Chill for at least 2 hours.

Per serving: 209 calories, 24 g carbohydrate, 8.5 g fat, 3.5 g fiber, 12 g protein, 6 mg cholesterol, 200 mg sodium. *Calories from fat: 36%.*

Apricot Dessert Bars

Makes 15 bars.

Filling
4 cups chopped fresh apricots
$^1/_3$ cup sugar
2 to 4 packets Sweet 'n Low
2 tablespoons Wondra flour

Base
Nonstick cooking spray
2 cups all-purpose or unbleached flour
$^1/_2$ cup sugar
3 to 6 packets Sweet 'n Low
$^1/_2$ teaspoon salt
$^1/_2$ teaspoon baking soda
3 tablespoons butter or margarine
$^1/_3$ cup nonfat cream cheese
2 tablespoons butter or margarine, melted
3 to 4 tablespoons low-fat buttermilk
$^2/_3$ cup flaked coconut
$^1/_4$ cup chopped pecans or walnuts

In medium saucepan, cook apricots over medium heat for a few minutes. Stir in sugar, 2 to 4 packets Sweet 'n Low (if you are sensitive to the aftertaste of artificial sweeteners, use the smaller amount), and Wondra flour. Continue to heat a couple more minutes or until nicely thickened; set aside.

Preheat oven to 400°. Coat bottom of 13-by-9-inch baking pan with nonstick cooking spray. In large bowl, combine flour, $1/2$ cup sugar, 3 to 6 packets Sweet 'n Low, salt, and baking soda. Using pastry blender, cut in 3 tablespoons butter and cream cheese. Drizzle melted butter or margarine and 3 tablespoons of buttermilk over the top and work in, using pastry blender. The mixture should be crumbly yet moist. Add coconut and pecans. Reserve $1^{1}/2$ cups of mixture. Press the remaining mixture in bottom of prepared pan. Bake for 8 minutes. Remove from oven. Spread apricot filling evenly over the crust. Sprinkle with remaining crumb mixture and bake an additional 12 to 15 minutes, or until top crust is golden brown. Cool. Cut into 15 bars.

Per bar: 193 calories, 31 g carbohydrate, 6.5 g fat, 2 g fiber, 4 g protein, 11 mg cholesterol, 193 mg sodium. *Calories from fat:* 30%.

Peanut Butter Oat Bran Bars

Makes 6 bars.

$1/2$ cup peanut butter
2 tablespoons lite pancake syrup
1 cup oat bran
$1/2$ cup Rice Krispies

Add peanut butter and pancake syrup to medium-size microwave-safe bowl. Microwave on High for $1^{1}/2$ to 2 minutes. Stir in oat bran and Rice Krispies. Press mixture into standard-size loaf pan. Chill for an hour. Cut into 6 bars.

Per serving: 195 calories, 22 g carbohydrate, 12 g fat, 5 g fiber (mostly soluble fiber), 9 g protein, 74 mg sodium. *Calories from fat:* 55%.

INDEX

Page numbers in *italics* refer to nutrition tables and lists.

abdominal obesity, 56, 57
acarbose (Precose), 12, 13–14
ACE inhibitors, 13
acesulfame-K, 28–29
aging, 47
albuminuria, 18, 19
alcohol
    blood glucose and, 31, 40
    calories and, 13
    diabetes complications and, 31, 48
    diabetes medications and, 13
    hypoglycemia and, 31
    insulin levels and, 30–31
    recommended limits on, 40
    triglycerides and, 31
Amaryl, 12
American Diabetes Association (ADA)
        recommendations
    carbohydrates, 20, 38–39, 76
    dietary cholesterol, 38–39
    fats, 37–38
    fiber, 39
    individualized diet plans, 36–37
    protein, 40–41
    sodium, 40
    sugar, 25–26, 38–39
amino acids, 13
angiotensin-converting enzyme (ACE)
        inhibitors, 13
antioxidants, 52–53
artificial sweeteners, 26–30, 153
aspartame, 27–28
aspirin, 13
atherosclerosis, 20, 23. *See also* heart
        disease
attitude, 65
avocados, 125

Beano, 21–22
beans, 21, 52, 54, 126–27
behavioral specialists, 15
blood cholesterol. *See* cholesterol,
        blood
blood glucose. *See* glucose, blood
blood pressure
    exercise and, 62, 63
    fiber and, 20
    preventing complications from, 48
    sodium and, 40
blood sugar. *See* glucose, blood
blood tests
    cholesterol, 11, 19–20
    glycohemoglobin, 11
    hemoglobin A1c, 13, 14
    lipids, 11, 19–20
    triglycerides, 11, 13, 19–20
bread, 110
breakfast
    recipes, 179–86
    tips, 133–36

calories
    alcohol and, 31
    artificial sweeteners and, 30
    burning, 59–60
    C-F-F Gram-Counting Plan and,
        78–79
    cutting, 42, 59, 60
    fat and, 18, 37, 38
    weight loss and, 36–37, 59
cancer prevention, 52–53, 126
canola oil, 22
carbohydrates
    absorption of, 43–45

carbohydrates *(cont'd)*
  balancing with fats, fiber, and
     protein, 18–20, 25, 38–39, 108,
     133–34
  blood glucose levels and, 18–20, 25,
     38–39, 44, 74
  C-F-F Gram-Counting Plan and,
     69–70, 74–76, 80–83
  complex, 25, 39
  diet high in, 19–20, 23–24, 39, 52,
     54, 127
  fats and, 18, 37, 38
  fiber and, 19–24, 52, 127, 133–34
  glycemic index and, 44–47,
     110–18
  insulin and, 12, 80–82
  lipids and, 20
  metabolism of, 12
  recommended amounts of, 19–20,
     38–39, 76, 80, 107–8
  simple, 25, 28
  sources of, 74
  sugar and, 25–26, 38–39
  triglycerides and, 19, 23, 24, 38, 54
carbohydrate-to-insulin ratio, 80–82
cardiovascular disease. *See* heart
     disease; stroke
cereals, 134–35
certified diabetes educators (CDEs), 8,
     9, 11
C-F-F Gram-Counting Plan
  Better Fast-Food Choices, *138–45*
  blood glucose and, 83–84
  Calculating C-F-F, *85–106*
  calories and, 78–79
  carbohydrates, 69–70, 74–76, 80–83
  combination foods, 83
  daily targets, 79–80
  fat, 70, 76–77, 80
  fiber, 70, 77–78
  insulin supplements and, 80–82
  Nutrition Facts label and, 73
  portion sizes and, 70–72

cholesterol, blood
  exercise and, 62, 63
  fiber and, 19–20, 21, 52, 77–78
  genetics and, 55
  HDL, 11, 23, 50, 51
  heart disease and, 38
  LDL, 11, 23, 50, 52, 55
  low-fat diets and, 55
  meal planning and, 64
  monounsaturated fats and, 22–23, 51
  polyunsaturated fats and, 23
  recommended levels of, 50
  saturated fats and, 22, 55
  testing of, 19–20, 49–50
  vitamin E and, 52
  VLDL, 50
cholesterol, dietary
  and blood cholesterol, 55
  foods high in, 51, 124
  heart disease and, 38
  and Mediterranean diet, 124
  recommended limits on, 22, 38, 107
combination foods, 83
complications of diabetes
  blood glucose levels and, 34, 35,
     47–48
  heart disease, 11, 31, 38, 48, 49
  high blood pressure, 48
  intensive therapy and, 34, 35
  nephropathy, 34, 48
  neuropathy, 34, 48
  renal disease, 13, 40–41
  retinopathy, 34, 48
  stroke, 48, 49
  table of, *48*
constipation, 21, 77
coronary artery disease. *See* heart
     disease
counseling for, 16

dehydration, 13
desserts
  as part of meals, 25

planning for, 120
recipes, 205–13
Diabetes Control and Complications
  Trial (DCCT), 34–36
diabetes management. *See also* meal
  planning; treatment plans
  blood glucose control and, 42–48,
    83–84
  intensive therapy for, 9, 34–37
  keys to, 7–8
  lifestyle changes for, 7, 37, 42, 49, 58
  self-care and, 7, 34
diabetic ketoacidosis, 13
diabetic retinopathy, 34, 48
diet diary, 108–10
dietitians, registered, 15
diet plans
  high-carbohydrate, 19–20, 23–24,
    39, 52, 54, 127
  high-fat, 23–24, 54
  high-fiber, 19–22, 52
  high-monounsaturated-fat, 23–24
  individualized, 14–15, 36–37
  low-carbohydrate, 39
  low-fat, 37–38, 50–51, 54, 55, 60
  low-glycemic-index, 46–47
  protein restriction, 18, 40
  for weight loss, 37–38, 58–62
digestion, 43–44, 59
dinner tips, 137

eating plans. *See* diet plans; meal
  planning
eggs, 135
electrolyte imbalance, 13
emergencies, 14
emotional eating, 120
endocrinologists, 15
entrée recipes, 193–205
Equal, 27–28
exchange system, 69
exercise
  benefits of, 62–63

diabetes complications and, 48, 62
diabetes management and, 7, 8, 42,
  62–64, 84
diet diary and, 108
insulin and, 62, 63
low-glycemic-index foods and, 111
planning for, 63–64
recommendations, 63
specialists, 8, 15, 64
for weight loss, 59, 62
exercise specialists, 8, 15, 64
eye problems, 34, 48

families
  counseling for, 16
  as health care team members, 16
  support from, 151
fast food, 137–45
Fast-Food Choices, Better, *138–45*
fat gene, 56–57
fats
  balancing carbohydrates with, 18–20
  blood glucose levels and, 18, 76,
    135
  calories and, 18, 37, 38
  C-F-F Gram-Counting Plan and, 70,
    76–77, 80
  diet high in, 23–24, 54
  diet low in, 37–38, 50–51, 54, 55,
    60
  foods low in, 164–65
  glycemic index and, 44
  heart disease risk and, 48, 49–51
  insulin and, 13
  lipid levels and, 38
  metabolism of, 13
  monounsaturated, 22–24, 38, 51,
    107–8 124–25
  no-sugar products and, 155
  polyunsaturated, 22, 23, 38, 107
  recommended amounts of, 37–38, 107
  saturated, 22, 38, 48, 50–51, 55,
    107, 124

fiber
  benefits of, 20, 77–78
  blood glucose and, 20–22, 77
  carbohydrates and, 19–24, 52, 127,
    133–34
  in cereals, 135
  C-F-F Gram-Counting Plan and, 70,
    77–78
  cholesterol and, 19–20, 21, 52,
    77–78
  glycemic index and, 45
  insulin requirements and, 21, 77
  lipid levels and, 39, 52, 77–78
  recommended amounts of, 21, 39,
    52, 78, 107, 127
  sources of, 20, 24, 127–33
  supplements, 39
fish, 51, 126
folate (folic acid), 53–54
food labels, 73, 153–54
free and almost-free foods
  recipes, 122–24
  using, 121
fructose, 44
fruits, 45, 126

garlic, 126
gluconeogenesis, 13
Glucophage, 12
glucose, blood
  alcohol and, 31, 40
  carbohydrates and, 18–20, 25,
    38–39, 44, 74
  carbohydrate-to-insulin ratio and,
    80–82
  controlling, 42–48, 83–84
  diabetes complications and, 34, 35,
    47–48
  digestion and, 43–44
  exercise and, 62–64
  fats and, 18, 76, 135
  fiber and, 20–22, 77
  glycemic index and, 44–47, 74
  glycohemoglobin testing of, 11

  high levels of, 13
  intensive insulin therapy and, 35
  ketoacidosis and, 13
  low-calorie sweeteners and, 30
  low levels of, 31, 36
  meal planning and, 64–65, 80–84,
    108–10
  monitoring, 7, 8, 14, 63–64, 108
  sugar and, 25
  "tight control" of, 9, 34–37
glycemic index
  factors affecting, 44–45
  guide to, 110
  insulin response and, 45, 111
  meal planning and, 45–47, 74,
    110–11
  purpose of, 44–45
  satiety and, 47
  "slow" meals and, 111
Glycemic Index of Foods, *112–18*
glycogen, 12
glycohemoglobin test, 11, 48

habits, changing, 150–51
HDL cholesterol
  dietary fats and, 23, 51
  increasing, 50
  testing of, 11
health care team
  building, 8–9, 15
  diet therapy and, 14–15
  emergencies and, 14
  exercise planning and, 8, 64
  families as members, 16
  first visit with, 9–10
  follow-up visits with, 11
  glucose monitoring instruction by,
    14
  medications and, 11–14
  members of, 8–9, 11, 15
  self-management and, 34
  specialists, 15
  tests and, 11
  "tight control" and, 9

heart attack, 37
heart disease
    alcohol and, 31, 48
    cholesterol and, 38
    exercise and, 48, 62
    fat and, 48, 49–51
    fiber and, 52
    folate and, 53
    genetics and, 54–55
    lipid levels and, 11, 49
    meal planning and, 64
    preventing, 48
    vitamin E and, 52–53
hemoglobin A1c, 13, 14
hepatic lipogenesis, 13
high-density lipoprotein. *See* HDL
    cholesterol
homocysteine, 53
Humalog, 12
hunger, 61, 119–20
hydrogenated oils, 51
hyperglycemia, 13
hypertension
    as diabetes complication, 48
    exercise and, 62, 63
    fiber and, 20, 40
hypoglycemia, 31, 36
hypoglycemics, oral, 12, 13

ice cream, 155, 159–61
insulin
    actions of, 12–13
    alcohol and, 30
    basal, 81
    carbohydrates and, 12, 80–82
    carbohydrate-to-insulin ratio,
        80–82
    C-F-F Gram-Counting Plan and,
        80–82
    exercise and, 62, 63
    fiber and, 21, 77
    glycemic index and, 45, 111
    intensive therapy with, 35
    oral hypoglycemics and, 13

    resistance, 12, 55, 56, 62
    response to food, 45
    supplements, 12, 35, 80–82
    weight loss with, 58–59
intensive therapy, 9, 34–37

ketoacidosis, 13
ketones, 13
ketosis, 13
kidney disease. *See* renal disease

lactose, 44
LDL cholesterol
    desirable levels of, 50
    dietary fats and, 23, 38
    genetics and, 55
    oxidation of, 23, 52
    testing of, 11
    vitamin E and, 52
lifestyle changes
    exercise, 42
    heart disease and stroke risk and, 49
    meal planning, 37, 42
    self-care and, 7
    weight loss, 42, 58
lipids, blood
    carbohydrates and, 20
    dietary fat and, 38
    exercise and, 62
    fiber and, 39, 52, 77–78
    garlic and, 126
    genetics and, 55
    glycemic index and, 46
    heart disease and, 11, 49–50
    normalizing, 42, 49–55
    testing of, 11, 49
lipolysis, 13
lipoprotein lipase, 13
low-density lipoprotein. *See* LDL
    cholesterol
lunch tips, 136–37

maltitol, 29
mannitol, 29, 153

meal planning. *See also* C-F-F Gram-
    Counting Plan; diet plans
    American Diabetes Association
        guidelines for, 36–41
    benefits of, 33–34, 82–83
    blood glucose and, 64–65, 80–84,
        108–10
    for breakfast, 133–36
    carbohydrates and, 19–20, 25–26,
        37–39, 74–76
    cholesterol levels and, 64
    diabetes management and, 7–8, 42
    diet diary for, 108–10
    for dinner, 137
    exercise and, 63–64
    fast food and, 137–38
    fats and, 23–24, 76–77
    glycemic index and, 45–47, 74,
        110–11
    for heart disease prevention, 64
    individualized, 14–15, 20, 24, 36–37
    issues to consider in, 36–37
    for lunch, 136–37
    portion sizes and, 25, 70–73, 137,
        146, 153
    small, frequent meals and, 64–65
    snacks and, 25, 119–21
    sugar and, 25–26
    systems, 69–70
    timing medication and, 119, 146
    triglycerides and, 36–37, 38, 54
    for weight loss, 37–38, 58–62
meal sizes, 64
mealtime tips
    breakfast, 133–36
    dinner, 137
    lunch, 136–37
    restaurants, 135–36, 145–46
measuring food, 71–72
meat, 124
medications for diabetes
    acarbose (Precose), 12, 13–14
    alcohol and, 13
    Amaryl, 12

    aspirin and, 13
    diet diary and, 108
    Glucophage, 12
    Humalog, 12
    insulin, 12, 35, 58–59, 80–82
    metformin, 12, 13
    oral hypoglycemics, 12, 13
    Rezulin, 12
    sulfonylureas, 12, 13
    timing with meals, 119, 146
Mediterranean diet, 124–27
Menu Items, Most Ordered, *146–50*
metabolism, 12–13
metformin, 12, 13
microalbuminuria, 19
monitoring, blood glucose
    diet diary and, 108
    exercise and, 63–64
    instructions from health care team,
        14
    as key to diabetes management, 7, 8
monounsaturated fats
    benefits of, 22–23, 51
    blood cholesterol and, 22–23, 51
    diet high in, 23–24, 124–25
    Mediterranean diet and, 124–25
    recommended amounts of, 107–8
    sources of, 22, 108, 125

National Cholesterol Education
        Program for Adults, 50
nausea, 14
nephrologists, 15
nephropathy, 34, 40–41, 48. *See also*
    renal disease
nerve damage, 34, 48
neuropathy, 34
NutraSweet, 27–29
nutrient analyses, 83
Nutrition Facts label, 73, 153–54

obesity. *See also* weight loss
    abdominal, 56
    fat gene and, 56–57

fiber and, 20–21
high-fat diet and, 38
measuring, 56, 57
stomach capacity and, 61–62
oils, 22, 51
olive oil, 22, 51, 125
omega-3 fatty acids, 51
ophthalmologists, 15
oral hypoglycemics, 12, 13
overeating, 61–62, 119–21

pasta, 110
pharmacists, 15
phenylalanine, 28
physical exams, 10
physicians
    exercise planning and, 64
    first visit with, 9–10
    follow-up visits with, 11
    as health care team members, 9, 15
    specialists, 15
    "tight control" and, 9
phytochemicals, 126
podiatrists, 15
polyunsaturated fats
    cholesterol and, 23
    monunsaturated versus, 22, 23
    recommended amounts of, 38, 107
portion sizes, 25, 70–73, 137, 146, 153
Precose (acarbose), 12, 13–14
protein
    balancing carbohydrates with, 18,
        19, 25, 133–34
    diabetes complications and, 48
    insulin and, 12–13
    metabolism of, 12–13
    recommended amounts of, 18–19,
        40–41, 107
    renal disease and, 18, 40–41
    sources of, 41
    in urine, 11, 18, 19
    vegetable, 19, 40, 41
psychologists, 15

recipes
    desserts, 205–13
    entrées, 193–205
    free and almost-free, 122–24
    list of, 177–79
    side dishes, 187–91
    snacks, 191–93
    to wake up to, 179–86
registered dietitians, 15
renal disease
    ACE inhibitors and, 13
    intensive therapy and, 34
    preventing, 48
    protein and, 18, 40–41
restaurant meals
    breakfast, 135–36
    fast-food, 137–45
    lunch, 136–37
    Most Ordered Menu Items, *146–50*
    tricks for, 145–46
retinopathy, 34, 48
Rezulin, 12

saccharin, 27, 29
sandwiches, 136–37
satiety, 47, 111, 119
saturated fats
    blood cholesterol and, 22, 55
    diabetes complications and, 48,
        50–51
    meat and, 124
    recommended limits on, 38, 107
self-management, 7, 34
serving sizes, 25, 70–73, 137, 146, 153
side-dish recipes, 187–91
small, frequent meals, 64–65
smoking, 48
snacks
    "free," 121
    insulin supplements and, 82
    overeating and, 119–21
    as part of meals, 25
    recipes, 191–93
sodium, 40, 48

sorbitol, 29, 30, 153
spouses, 151
starches. *See* carbohydrates
stomach capacity, 61–62
stress, 63, 120
stroke, 37, 48, 49, 53
sucrose, 25, 44
sugar, blood. *See* glucose, blood
sugar, dietary
    alternatives to, 26–30
    American Diabetes Association
        recommendations for, 25–26,
        38–39
    blood glucose levels and, 25
    carbohydrates and, 25–26, 38–39
    diabetes complications and, 48
    fructose, 44
    glycemic index and, 44–45
    lactose, 44
    Less-Sugar-Added Products, *162–64*
    meal planning and, 25–26
    No-Sugar-Added Products, *155–62*
    no-sugar products, 152–53, 155
    portion sizes of, 25
sugar alcohols, 29–30, 153
Sugar Twin, 29
sulfonylureas, 12, 13
Sunette, 28–29
supplements
    fiber, 39
    insulin, 12, 35, 80–82
    vitamin E, 52–53
support groups, 9, 15, 151
sweeteners, artificial, 26–30, 153
Sweet'n Low, 29
Sweet One, 28–29

*Taste vs. Fat: Rating the Low-Fat and
    Fat-Free Foods* (Magee), 153
"tight control," 9, 34–37
treatment plans
    diet therapy and, 14–15

    individualized, 7, 8, 14–15, 34
    intensive, 9, 34–37
    medications and, 11–14
    reviewing, 11
triglycerides
    alcohol and, 31
    carbohydrates and, 19, 23, 24, 38,
        54
    exercise and, 62
    fat metabolism and, 13
    fiber and, 20
    insulin and, 13
    recommended levels of, 50
    testing of, 11

urine, protein in, 11, 18, 19

vegetables, 126
very low density lipoprotein (VLDL),
    50
vitamin E, 52–53
vomiting, 14

weight loss
    amount needed, 17, 31–32
    aspartame and, 27
    benefits of, 56
    diabetes complications and, 48
    for diabetes management, 42, 48,
        55–56
    exercise and, 59, 62
    fat gene and, 56–57
    fiber, 20–21
    high-monounsaturated-fat diet and,
        24
    with insulin, 58–59
    low-fat diet and, 37–38, 60
    meal planning for, 37–38, 58–62
    stomach capacity and, 61–62
    strategies for, 58, 59

xylitol, 29

ABOUT THE AUTHOR

Elaine Magee, M.P.H., R.D., is a Registered Dietitian who emphasizes good-tasting, convenient food along with good nutrition. For two years, she performed the *Light Cooking* segment for the KSBW-TV (NBC) midday news in the Salinas/Santa Cruz/Gilroy area, and she has appeared on both national and local television. Her column, "The Recipe Doctor," is featured in the *Contra Costa Times* (a Knight-Ridder paper).

As a consumer nutrition expert, she was a consultant to a highly successful twenty-six-store supermarket chain in California for six years. She has also consulted for local and national food companies such as Dole Packaged Foods, as well as for government agencies, including the California Department of Health "5 a Day" programs. She has been a featured speaker at health conferences, has written practical consumer pamphlets, and has developed several quick and healthy recipes that have won awards in California and been distributed nationally. She has written eleven cookbooks and books on nutrition, including *Eat Well for a Healthy Menopause,* also from Wiley.

Elaine Magee lives in northern California with her husband and two daughters, ages four and six.